TWO CENTURIES OF STRIFE

HEALTH WARS IN NEW SOUTH WALES

T0363159

BY DAVID G. THOMAS

Atlantis Books

Dedicated to the memory of PETER TREBILCO, OAM
'78-er'
Long-time teacher and colleague in our School.
Friend to so many in it.

First published in Australia in 2020
by Atlantis Books
48 Ross Street, Glebe NSW 2037
www.littlesteps.com.au
www.atlantisbooks.com.au

Text copyright © 2020 David G. Thomas

A Catalogue-In-Publication entry for this book is available from
the National Library of Australia.

ISBN: 978-1-922358-20-2

Designed by Nina Nielsen
Printed in China
10 9 8 7 6 5 4 3 2 1

CONTENTS

INTRODUCTION

Health and healing have always been of fundamental concern to human beings. Equally fundamental is that there has always been disagreement and indeed conflict over how best health can be maintained and healing effected. A typical example of such conflict can be found in the records of both the past and the present in even a relatively small entity such as the State of New South Wales in Australia.

That State of course, owes its existence to the invasion and settlement of south-eastern Australia by British migrants which began in 1788. These invaders ignored the thinking of the original Aboriginal inhabitants about health and healing and instead imported a multitude of often conflicting health epistemologies from their 'mother countries' in the British isles.

As their new society organised itself, its health modalities formed themselves into rival camps. On the one hand there was what could be termed the formal health system, recognised by governments and operated by those with recognised qualifications granted by institutions of higher learning. On the other hand, there was an informal system in which practice was open to anyone who chose to call themselves a healer and which was used initially by the majority of the population who distrusted and therefore eschewed the formal system. That over the next century-and-a-half of the proponents of both the formal and informal camps were so hostile and attacked each other with such ferocity that their conflict can justifiably be described as a 'war'.

The enormous, indeed epochal changes in the understandings of both health and healing which took place from the mid-19th century onwards enabled the formal system to become dominant the world over. Still, the informal system which became known as 'alternative/complementary' medicine, continued in vigorous existence and indeed began to strengthen its position from the second half of the 20th century onwards. During these decades the 'war' between the two camps continued unabated.

This work sets out to trace the course of that war and in so doing, demonstrates that it involved not only medical issues, but has also been strongly influenced and indeed determined by economic, social and particularly political developments in the State of NSW.

What emerges and will be demonstrated in this work is that one of the most important factors governing the fortunes of the conflicting sides was not simply their medical efficacy, but governmental recognition embodied in the form of legal regulation. Rather than being seen as a burden, such regulation seemingly confers an official guarantee of trustworthiness and reliability on the suppliers of a medical modality and was and is therefore enormously valuable to the practitioners of that modality.

For that reason, gaining the recognition implied by governmental regulation was as eagerly sought after by both sides of the war as was the legendary Holy Grail of ancient times. In this respect, NSW is not unique but is rather typical of other entities in and around the world. For that reason the developments recorded in this volume have relevance to other jurisdictions in which there have been and still are similar conflicts between competing medical modalities.

WHY NEW SOUTH WALES?

To answer that question it needs first of all to be pointed out that in Australia, the medico/political struggles being analysed have taken place as much as on a State as on a national level. Australian States of course, are the successors to the six colonies established in the roughly half-century following the British invasion/settlement of 1788. Each of the colonies was founded at different times for different reasons and developed different polities and politics before they grudgingly agreed to form the federated Commonwealth of

Australia in 1901. The federal form of that Commonwealth meant that its component States continued to operate as semi-sovereign political entities which had primary oversight over, among other things, the health care field.

This situation continued long after 1901: there was no federal Department of Health until 1921 and both before and after that time the colonies/States developed distinctive and sometimes idiosyncratic modes of dealing with health issues which are worth recording in their own right. Moreover, while in time the issues covered by this book did become nation rather than merely State-wide, in 2008 it was New South Wales which took the lead on the issue of introducing the Holy Grail of regulation into the field of alternative/complementary medical practice which, as detailed in Chapter 1, was first raised in the deliberations of its Legislative Council in 1838. On that basis it is argued, rather than looking at Australia as a whole, fuller understandings of the issues can equally well be gained by starting at the level of the individual States and particularly the State of New South Wales (NSW), and then extrapolating these findings to the rest of the country.

TERMINOLOGY

To avoid the endless terminological wrangling described for example by Coulter and Willis in the early 21st century, the different and often conflicting medical modalities dealt with in this work are designated as 'Mainstream Medicine' (MM) and 'UnConventional Medicine' (UCM). The acronym MM is used to denote 'official' medicine in the sense that grounded in academic or tertiary training, it is recognised and supported by governments and thus given official legitimation. It covers those therapeutic activities served by the medical profession and all its branches and also hospital and ancillary health institutions used at various times (including the present) by the majority of the population. While the term 'allopathic' medicine could have been and indeed was used to describe these kinds of therapies for the earlier part of the period covered by this work, it tends to be outdated and therefore obscure.

For its part, the acronym 'UCM' denotes those therapies contemporaneously described as 'complementary medicine' or 'alternative medicine', often denoted by the acronym CAM. The use those terms is avoided because they have been applied to these modalities only in very recent times - in fact, less than a quarter of the timespan being covered in this work. For the greater part of that period there was no collective noun for them, apart from the term 'fringe medicine' which was used by some in the mid-20th century but which never caught-on to any great extent. To apply the terms 'alternative' or 'complementary' medicine during the first 175 years of the 'Two Centuries of Strife' under discussion, would be anachronistic, while the term 'unconventional medicine' denoted by the acronym UCM can appropriately be applied to these modalities during all the time periods covered.

CHAPTER 1

Battleground New South Wales

What is a medical practitioner? The members of the Legislative Council of New South Wales urgently needed an answer to that question. The year was 1838 and they were mulling over the establishment of the first Coronial Court in the Colony of New South Wales. The functioning of that Court was dependent on the testimonies of legally recognised medical practitioners, but at the time, there was there was no universally accepted definition of any such functionary.

Still, the Council had the benefit of an exploration of this issue in the form of an earlier failed 'Medical Practice Act' which had sought to lay down that a medical practitioner was a man (definitely no women at that time) who could prove that he was '… a Doctor or Bachelor of Medicine of some University or a Physician or Surgeon, or admitted as such by some College of Physicians or Surgeons in Great Britain or Ireland…'.[1]

That definition excluded the large number of people claiming to be medical practitioners, who while lacking any such qualifications, were active in NSW at the time. In the words of Dr James Russell, a surgeon who testified before a Select Committee on the Medical Practice Act, these included:

Midwives, Herbalists, Cuppers, Barbers, Electricians, Galvanisers, Dentists, Farriers, Veterinary Surgeons, Village Wisemen and Cow Leeches.[2]

Russell asserted that these practitioners (some of whom even in his day would surely have been thought bizarre), should be allowed to practice unhindered, but most of the dozen other medical men who also testified disagreed. One such was Dr James Bowman, 'late inspector general of Colonial Hospitals' who asserted that since unqualified practitioners were guilty of 'public mischief', not only would it be wrong to grant them any official recognition, but that they should 'undoubtedly' be prohibited from practising and that such prohibition should be 'absolute'.[3]

Those arguments put forward in 1838 help to set the scene for the 'war' between those types of therapy and orthodox medical practice in the State of New South Wales (NSW) which has raged for close on 200 years. While that conflict has been evident in many different fields, what is important about the arguments of 1838 is that they took place in the official decision-making forum of the Colony. That in turn indicated that the fortunes and future of the conflicting medical therapies specified in the 1838 debate would be crucially dependent on their recognition or non-recognition by NSW governments in the form of medical regulation.

Any idea that medical regulation is an inconsequential issue is belied by the way it has been as eagerly sought as the original, fabled Holy Grail. Yet of course medical regulation is nothing like as mythical as that original. As this study will show, its perceived benefits have always been coveted and pursued by major interest groups including those needing or likely to need health care services – which in fact means the population at large - and also the practitioners of medical therapies of whatever kind in the State of NSW and beyond. That these groups have sought for and fought over medical regulation with such ferocity throughout the past two centuries means that it is not over-dramatic to call their contests a 'war'.

Medical practice and practitioners

One of the most important starting points of this account of the 'war' between Mainstream Medicine (MM) and UnConventional

Medicine (UCM) in New South Wales is that MM has always been the official modality recognised and used by governments. Even before the British invasion/settlement of January 1788, the government attempted to provide for the health needs of the 1,400 convicts transported to Australia by appointing nine doctors to the vessels of that 'First Fleet'. Despite the doubtful qualifications of most, they continued to serve as officially-appointed medical practitioners after the cargo of convicts had been dumped at Sydney Cove. Moreover one of the first government 'structures' erected after the landing was a tent-hospital which continued to serve this purpose until a stone-built hospital provided by the Colonial government was taken into use in 1816. This was Australia's first permanent hospital and although much altered it still stands next to the State Parliament close to Sydney's city centre.

Although strongly shaped by class factors, governmental recognition and support for MM was ostensibly due to its research efforts and training regimes being university-based, even though that training tended to draw on ancient 'humoral' theories of health and disease dating back to before the time of Hippocrates - sometimes called 'the Father of Medicine' - in the 3rd century BCE. In terms of humoral understandings, disease was a result of imbalances between the four 'humors' in the body – black bile, yellow bile, phlegm and the blood. Attempts to correct those imbalances led to the drawing of oceans of blood (a procedure known as venesection) from millions of patients for over 2,000 years. While during the 19th century such 'therapy' and the ideas behind it were in the course of being discarded by the teachers and practitioners of MM in favour of newly-sprung scientific medicine, the radical changes in their medical epistemology did nothing to change and in fact probably re-inforced their strongly negative views of UCM, which they labeled as 'quack medicine'.

Yet having been abundantly present in the 'mother-country' of Britain for hundreds of years and, as is clear from the discussions leading to the establishment of the first NSW Coronial Court in 1838, 'quacks' were bound to make an early appearance as successive waves of British immigrants joined the invasion/settlement of NSW.[4] Of course Indigenous Australians, during their plus/minus 60,000 years of occupation of Australia prior to its colonization, had developed their own epistemologies of health and healing which are described in some detail by Martyr in her authoritative *Paradise of Quacks*, although she also asserts that 'the traditions of Aboriginal medicine were abruptly displaced by the arrival of Europeans.'[5] While very probably that process was nothing like as abrupt as she claims, certainly there is no evidence of any attempt to systematize Aboriginal health practices or organise its practitioners and neither played any role in the 'war' between MM and UCM being described in this volume.

Later in the 19th century, the list of non-orthodox, that is UCM practitioners active in the colonialist population would have looked rather different to that put forward by Dr James Russell in the 1838 discussions on the establishment of the Coronial Court. According to Martyr, such a list would have included practitioners of ancient therapies such as herbalism and naturopathy as well as the newer modalities of electrotherapy, phrenology, hydrotherapy, magnetism, galvanism, and psychopathy.[5]

Not included in that list are relatively recently emergent therapies whose progenitors, in the eyes of their followers anyway, enjoyed a semi-messianic status. These included the German founder of homeopathy, Samuel Hahnemann (1755-1843), who asserted that because 'like treats like', disease could be remedied by treating it with special preparations which incorporated elements of the disease itself in a highly diluted form.[6] Chiropractic was and is a therapeutic system founded by an American physician, Daniel D. Palmer (1845-1913), based on the idea that physical pathologies are due to misalignments in the skeletal system which can be cured by manipulation of that system to bring it back into its proper alignment.[7] Osteopathy, likewise founded by Andrew T. Still (1828-1917), treats physical disorders by seeking to restore correct relationships between bones, muscles and connective tissues and often includes chiropractic-like manipulation of skeletal structures.

Moreover, as a result of closer contact with and immigration from Asia in the 20th century, Traditional Chinese Medicine and its offshoot, acupuncture, were added to UCM practice in Australia as a whole and NSW in particular.[8] Among the other curative systems developed later in the 20th century were aromatherapy, Bowen therapy, iridology, kinesiology, reiki and rolfing – although this list is by no means exhaustive. Due to their multiplicity, no attempt is made here to describe in detail the widely differing epistemologies of each of those listed above. However, one feature common to all and which set them apart from MM, is that their claims to validity were and are based on successful practical outcomes of their treatments rather than on scientifically derived knowledge.

A typical example of that is acupuncture, the practice of which consists of the insertion of fine needles into 'meridians' running through the body to produce a curative effect on various maladies. However, although large numbers of both practitioners and patients of acupuncture cite definite cures of various conditions, extensive research, scientific and otherwise, has failed to find any physical evidence of meridians in any one of the huge number of bodies, alive and dead, which have been investigated in this quest.[9]

Like acupuncture, each of the other therapies mentioned above was based on its own unique epistemology which, because being far removed from the official epistemologies of MM, enjoyed neither academic or as a consequence, governmental recognition or regulation in NSW until the late 20th century. Despite that, the services of practitioners of unconventional therapies were widely used in the 19th century. A leading scholar of NSW medical history Dr Peter Lloyd has noted that 'some of the more prominent quacks and irregular healers enjoyed a level of patronage and popularity of which many of their qualified counterparts would have been envious.'[10] Another prominent medical writer Prof Evan Willis points to the fierceness of the struggle between MM and UCM when he states: 'The homeopaths saw themselves as pioneers, as founders of a new paradigm of medicine...' and that '[t]hrough the 1870s and 1880s the controversy between homeopathy and allopathy [MM] raged in newspapers and journals'.[11]

Yet the scope of UCM usage cannot be encompassed by the practices listed here. It will be argued shortly that what also needs to be taken into account are a great number and range of informal practices such as those mentioned by Wannan in his *Folk Medicine. A Miscellany of Old Cures and Remedies in Australia* in which, based on his firsthand experience of rural life, he reported that

> ...the chief reason for the general avoidance of doctors in country areas, except when circumstances made it imperative to rely on their help, was that most folk in the pioneering era had learned to rely on the efficacy of their own home-prepared concoctions and cures, aided by ... store remedies and concoctions and patented specifics ... for many Australians, down to the period of the 1920s, a physician was generally thought of being the 'last resort'. It was the local chemist ... who was looked upon as the important man of medicine.[12]

As will be related, the suspicion of and often hostility to the medical profession among a wide segment of the population, chiefly those in the working classes, continued well into the 20th century.

Although UCM was being practised both before and after the outset of the white invasion/settlement in NSW, the proportion of the population who were using it during the next 100-odd years is unknown. Official statistics show the settler population had more than quadrupled from 357,978 in 1861 to 1,364,590 in 1900[13], but there were no official population measurements which might have recorded data relating to medical practice and beliefs.

One of the nearest indications of the strength of UCM can be gleaned from an unofficial source, Ludwig Bruck's *Australian Medical Directory* published in 1883 which listed the names of 526 UCM practitioners throughout Australia, 183 of them in NSW.[14] Although this was a miniscule figure compared to the 1,275 medically qualified practitioners who, according to Bruck, were active in the Colony at the time, it can be argued on the basis of Wannan's claims in his *Folk Medicine* quoted above, that the strength and following of UCM can never be deduced simply from the number of its practitioners and as will be argued later, this is as true of the 21st century as it was of the 19th. Moreover, that fierce contests between MM and UCM quickly developed in the Colony, indicates that the proponents of either side never saw UCM as the small and inconsequential phenomenon as the numbers of its practitioners recorded by Bruck might seem to suggest.

The early medical/epistemological dimensions of those contests have been very well and comprehensively covered by authors such as Martyr and Pensabene.[15] This work however, sets out to demonstrate that the conflict has been fought out in the political as much as in the medical sphere and focuses on how political factors and the actions of governments formed a major part of the health 'wars' between mainstream and complementary/alternative medicine in NSW.

The drive for medical regulation

One of the first pieces of legislation relating to health in NSW, the Medical Witnesses Act of 1838, was a corollary to that Act which established the Coronial Court in the same year. The Medical Witnesses Act was passed not as a regulatory measure, but merely to ensure that the physicians summoned to give evidence in Coronial Inquests were in possession of recognised medical qualifications. The vetting of those qualifications was placed in the hands of a Medical Board created by the Act, the members of which were appointed by the Legislative Council. It was the first such Board to be established anywhere in the world (although that claim is disputed by the State of Tasmania) and was charged with the maintenance of a Medical Register containing the names of physicians who could be summoned to give evidence at Inquests.

It should be emphasised that the 1838 Medical Witnesses Act was not a regulatory measure and did nothing to change the situation in NSW, where medical practice was a 'free-for-all' in which anyone, whatever their qualifications or lack of them, could claim to be a physician and make a living out of medical practice. That situation remained unchanged for over 60 years after 1838, as was affirmed by Dr Henry McLaurin, the chancellor of the University of Sydney, when he told a Parliamentary Select Committee in 1888 that in NSW: 'Anyone could practice medicine and advertise themselves as a doctor of medicine or as the holder of other medical qualifications'[16] including 'those who had no medical training whatsoever'. The only effect the Medical Witnesses Act might have had on such bogus practitioners was that their lack of qualifications might preclude them from giving evidence at a coronial inquest which, since that chore was unpaid, they would very likely have declined to do anyway.

The advent of medical regulation

Medical regulation, in terms of which only those with recognised medical qualifications could legally practice medicine, had been first introduced in Britain in the form of the Medical Practitioners' Act of 1858. That legal precedent was followed throughout the rest of the 19th century by the Australian colonies (although not to NSW as we shall see) to remedy uncontrolled and therefore seemingly dangerous medical practice. This was in line with the relatively new idea that governments should act to protect the health of their citizens which was displacing the old notion that the health of the citizenry was the private responsibility of individuals and families. The change was partly due to the upper and middle classes of Western societies becoming wealthier and experiencing rising standards of living. That development resulted, in the words of the great German sociologist Max Weber who saw this happening all around him in the late 19th and early 20th centuries, in an 'increasing need for order and protection in all fields'.[17] He might have added this was particularly true of the medical field, as can be seen for instance in a petition containing 1,360 signatures which was presented to the NSW government in March 1876. It claimed that the petitioners

...have hitherto been deprived of legal protection from injury and maltreatment in sickness, in consequence of there not being any Statute to restrain the fraud and imposture which is now extensively carried on throughout New South Wales by a class of persons professing to be duly qualified practitioners in the art and science of medicine and surgery, but who are in reality impostors, possessing no recognised qualifications whatever. That, in consequence of there being at present no such Act of Parliament in this Colony, we, your Petitioners, would respectfully pray a Medical Bill be brought before Parliament which would assimilate the laws with regard to the medical profession to those now in force in the United Kingdom [18]

The reference in the last line was to the British Medical Practitioners' Act, a precedent rapidly adopted in other jurisdictions around the world which passed legislation that not only laid down the qualifications required of physicians given the legal right to practice medicine, but also imposed penalties on any doctor who was found to have misbehaved egregiously, most particularly by being addicted to alcohol or drugs. (In Britain, committing adultery and performing abortions were seen to be equally heinous offences for over a century after the passing of the Medical Practitioners' Act of 1858[19]). The penalty of being 'struck off', that is, of having their name removed from the Medical Register and therefore forbidden to practice – was an economic death sentence for any doctor who relied on medical practice for their income.

An important point is that the powers specified in Medical Practitioners' Acts were not directly exercised by government but were delegated to controlling bodies composed of government-appointed physicians. In Britain this body was called the 'General Medical Council' (GMC), but in NSW there was ready-made institution in the form of the Medical Board set up in 1838. In the early to mid-19th century medical boards of this kind were novel entities and although they were appointed by governments and operated in terms of laws passed by governments, they were not seen to be accountable to government or in fact to anybody or anyone but themselves. That put a great deal of power into the hands of physicians and indeed it was this autonomy that in pure sociological terms, conferred on them the exalted status of 'profession'. As we shall see, other health-related occupations such as nursing, dentistry, pharmacy and optometry – and in time also UCM modalities - also lusted after this 'Holy Grail' of governmentally-recognised and supported professional status, the attraction of which became even more powerful after the members and all other expenses of professional registration boards began to be paid by government from the mid-20th century onwards.

Medical regulatory innovations were one aspect of one of the most remarkable although unremarked developments in human history – the enormous expansion of government and of governmental regulation, in the 19th and early 20th centuries. In the words of Stephen Drucker, in a famous article entitled 'The Sickness of Government,' he asserted that populations

> ...especially in the developed countries, were hypnotized by government. We were in love with and saw no limits to its abilities, or to its good intentions. ... Anything that anyone felt needed doing during this period was to be turned over to government - and this, everyone seemed to believe, made sure that the job was already done. [20]

Illustrative of Drucker's contention is that during the 19th century, government expenditure as a percentage of gross national product (GNP) increased from 15 per cent to 47 per cent in the United Kingdom, 10 per cent to 45 per cent in Germany and 5 per cent to 34 per cent in the United States. Although there are no comparable figures for Australia as a whole, in NSW the growth of the government bureaucracy was probably even faster. Thus, while between 1860 and 1895 the population of NSW grew by 262% (from 348,546 to 1,262,270), between 1859 and 1894 the number of public servants increased from 843 to 32,722 - a rise of 3,793% .[21]

Servicing the needs of growing populations was important for the political arm of governments to enable them, among other things, to extend and defend their electoral fortunes. In this respect, attempting to safeguard the safety of populations by means of regulation was a priority for governments. However, while notionally designed to promote public safety, regulation in especially the medical field also had the potential to 'ring-fence' qualified medical practitioners against economic competition by unqualified practitioners and thus constituted what Weber described as 'economic closure'.[22] In other words, governmental regulation seemingly guaranteed the economic monopoly for those with the right qualifications.

This was one reason why the institution of medical regulation at that time was vitally important to the medical profession. The operation of the Medical Witnesses Act of 1838 and subsequent amendments, gives a crucial insight into the motivations of this group. But what first needs to be noted is that the Medical Board set up in terms of that Act was a weak body. As noted earlier, its main task was to check the validity of the qualifications presented by those who applied to have their names on the Medical Register. However, as chairman of the Board, Sir Arthur Renwick lamented in Parliament in 1880:

> ...the powers of the Board ... did not admit of a determination whether any gentlemen who presented for registration, were really and properly the possessors of the documents they showed or qualified to practice. ... Several applicants for registration had no doubt foresworn themselves and were now practicing in the Colony.[23]

Renwick's last sentence shows clearly that doctors, whether bona fide or bogus, were very keen to get their names on the Medical Register because that implied legal recognition of their right to practise. Although this was not the case since the Register established in 1838 merely contained the names of those doctors who could be called on to give evidence at coronial inquests, none the less having their name on the Register implied governmental recognition of an individual doctor's qualifications and was a useful means of attracting a clientele and therefore had an economic value. That the numbers on the Medical Register rose from 6 in 1839 to 1,906 in 1889,[24] indicates that from the outset, any kind of official governmental endorsement of a doctor's qualifications was seen as a crucial asset, economically as much as in any other respect. That helps to explain why members of the medical profession and other therapeutic organisations strove so mightily to attain the Grail of full governmental regulation because that would emphatically and legally establish their exclusive right to practice in their field.

The benefits deriving from governmental recognition can be even more clearly seen from the record of the Medical Board the membership of which swelled from five in 1838 to 12 in 1900. Such membership betokened that an individual had been recognised as a leader in the medical profession and in fact in the colonial community as a whole – an even greater asset in attracting clientele or when seeking appointment to paid governmental or academic positions.

The exalted standing of the membership was evident from the outset, the first president appointed in 1838 being Dr J.V. Thomson, who was already Deputy Inspector-General of Hospitals. The other members were Dr J. Dobie, a surgeon with the Royal Navy who was to become a member of the legislature, Dr J. Robertson who was later to join the staff of the University of Sydney, as did Dr C. Nicholson who was also a member of the legislature. Finally there was a Dr. F. Wallace who had been trained in Edinburgh and after living in Sydney for six years, had become close to the local medical establishment.[24] These Board members were not paid but for reasons stated, willingly accepted their appointments to the MRB. Despite the Board's lack of any significant regulatory power during its first sixty years of existence, it was later granted a degree of power and autonomy unmatched by any other NSW government instrumentality throughout most of the 20th century.

This point can be supported by a short foray into the history of public administration in NSW and indeed in the rest of the world. The Medical Board constituted an early, indeed perhaps the earliest example of what may be called the 'expert co-optation principle'. When it established the Board in 1838, the government of the day, lacking anyone within its ranks who had any medical expertise, co-opted the medical 'experts' named above to perform the specialised function of checking the credentials of those who wished to have their names inscribed on the Medical Register. The same principle of expert co-optation was applied to cope with the enormous expansion of governmental activities in the later 19th century, when non-governmental people with expertise in or at least knowledge of a wide variety of fields, were co-opted to carry out governmental activities in bodies known as 'statutory authorities'. Today in NSW there are so many statutory authorities - ranging from the Sydney Opera House Trust to the Wild Dog Destruction Board - that it is difficult to ascertain their exact number. These bodies differed from the Medical Board in that they were attached to government departments and required each year to produce for the Parliament an annual report on their activities and finances.

Having been established long before statutory authorities were thought of, (they began to be introduced only in the 1880s) the Medical Board was never attached even to health departments and was never required to produce annual reports. In other words, the Medical Board was established as a wholly unaccountable administrative entity and remained that way between 1838 and 1987 – close on a century-and-a-half. That status, which reflected the exalted social status conferred on the medical profession especially by the upper classes, was to have far-reaching consequences, as will be demonstrated later in this work.

The Parliamentary battlefront

That governmental recognition of the right of a physician to practice medicine highlights the fact that the debates and decisions of legislative bodies in NSW were a crucial factor in the war between MM and UCM in the State. In turn, the way decisions were taken in NSW legislative bodies demands an understanding of their structure and the way these bodies functioned. On that score, the first important point to note is that the appointed Legislative Council, which in 1838 had established the NSW Coronial Court and passed the Medical Witnesses Act, continued in existence until 1856, when along with other Australian Colonies, New South Wales was granted responsible government. That meant that all but ultimate control of the Colony was devolved on its new Parliament. That Parliament was to become one of the chief battlegrounds between UCM and MM and to understand why, we first need to note that it was established as a bi-cameral legislature with an Upper House, the Legislative Council, the members of which were appointed by the Governor, and an elected Lower House, known as the Legislative Assembly. All legislation had to be passed by both Houses before it could become law.

The Upper House, the Legislative Council, was modelled on the House of Lords in Britain, its officially stated purpose being to constitute 'a safe, revising, deliberative and conservative element between the Lower House and Her Majesty's representatives'.[25] R.S. Parker, one of the leading scholars of NSW Parliamentary history, asserts that 'the nominee Council was conservative in practice, and generally in political complexion and action'.[26] In other words, one purpose of the Upper House was to act as a check on the wilder populist spirits of the Lower House but also betokened that it represented the interests of the upper, ruling class in the Colony.

This House consistently supported and voted for the introduction of medical regulation in NSW. In other words, it heavily favoured MM. Which is not surprising, seeing that one occupational grouping present in strength in the Upper House were leading medical practitioners such as Dr Sir Henry McLaurin and Dr Sir Arthur Renwick, both of whom served as Chancellors of the University of Sydney at various times. Another notable was Dr Richard Bowker, who served as both an elected member of the Lower House and later, as a nominated member of the Upper House.

But among the most formidable members and in many ways the leader of this group was Dr John Creed, a medical practitioner who had become a full-time politician; he was implacably opposed to UCM and worked relentlessly to strengthen the political power of the medical profession. This group or elite stood above the general run of medical practitioners, their status being reflected by their appointments to the Medical Board, as honoraries to major hospitals, to advisory positions in government and through their connections to what was then the only university in NSW, the University of Sydney, either as members of the Faculty of Medicine or as examiners.[27]

This elite formed the spearhead of MM in battles over medical regulation during the last decades of the 19th century and they exercised a long-lasting influence far beyond the confines of the Parliament. They were the driving force, for instance, in the formation of the NSW chapter of British Medical Association in 1878, the forerunner of the Australian Medical Association. Sir Arthur Renwick was its first president while Dr Creed was the first editor of its journal *The Australasian Medical Gazette*, forerunner to the *Medical Journal of Australia*. As Lloyd points out, unremitting hostility to 'quackery', otherwise UnConventional Medicine (UCM), was one of the more frequently occurring issues in its pages.[28]

For its part, the Lower House of the Parliament, the Legislative Assembly, was an elected body, the members of which were initially mostly drawn from the middle classes[27], although the payment of members after 1889 made it possible for more working class representatives to enter the Parliament.[28] One result of that change which is important to the overall argument of this book, is that one basis for the differences of between MM and UCM at that stage was an economic one. The middle and lower classes represented in the Lower House patronised and supported the collective interests of UCM practitioners because in that era the services of doctors were much more expensive than those of UCM practitioners. Thus the medical profession, whose interests were represented in the Upper House, got only meagre support from the middle and working classes and their representatives in the Lower House. The majority in this House, as will be recorded in the next chapter, consistently rejected the introduction of medical regulation. Thus the two Houses in the Parliament came to embody not only economically-based class differences but also the medical conflicts in NSW with the Upper House championing the cause of MM and the Lower House, that of UCM.

What may seem to be an inconsequential feature of that Parliament and the Lower House in particular, but which was in fact, crucially important in the war between UCM and MM in NSW, is that for over 50 years after its establishment there were no political parties and therefore no 'party discipline' in the Parliament. In terms of the unwritten edicts of party discipline, all members of a party were and are obliged to vote with their party on every issue, irrespective of their personal feelings or opinions. Any member who fails to vote with the party is disciplined by being expelled from the party – a political death sentence carried out at the next election when the party will turn the full weight of its financial and organisational power against the rebellious member to ensure that they lose their seat.

The lack of party discipline meant that every vote in the 19th century NSW Parliament was a free or conscience vote, members voting for or voting down every piece of legislation depending on their personal opinions or principles. However democratically admirable that may seem, the result in NSW was that its governments were unstable because of their inability to rely on any consistent bloc of support to get their legislation passed. Their failure on that score very often meant the governments had to resign, which accounts for the fact that in the first 50 years of responsible government in NSW, two-thirds of all legislation presented to the Parliament by the governments of the day failed to pass while governments regularly fell after being defeated, particularly in Lower House votes.[28] Notable among the failed pieces of legislation over the next half-century were Medical Practitioners' Bills which sought to ensure the safety of medical practice in the State by means of regulation modelled on the British Medical Practice Act.

The golden rule of tertiary training

While it was probably not obvious at the time and indeed is not so even today, the 1838 Medical Witnesses Act can be seen as a 'starter's gun' in a race for societal legitimacy between MM and UCM, the outcome of which would by no means have been certain at that time. The failure of that Act to define who or what constituted a 'legally qualified Medical Practitioner', gave rise to the discussion reported in the introductory chapter of this work, which led to the passing of another Act, in June 1838 to be precise, '… to define the qualifications of Medical Witnesses at Coroners' Inquests and Inquiries held before Justices of the Peace in the Colony of NSW' (2 Victoria No. 22). It is worthwhile repeating the terms of this clause of the Act in full because it defined a legally qualified practitioner as one who

> …is a Doctor or Bachelor of Medicine of some University or a Physician or Surgeon licensed or admitted as such by some College of Physicians or Surgeons in Great Britain or Ireland or is a Member of the Company of Apothecaries of London or who is or has been a Medical Officer duly appointed and confirmed of Her Majesty's land or sea service.

(This last-named qualification remained in force for the next hundred years.) Those terms of the 1838 Act meant that MM started its race for societal legitimacy with a huge advantage in that its training was based on tertiary university education. This was despite the fact that the medical knowledge taught at that time still drew on the ancient humoral approaches described earlier in this chapter. While such theories and medical practices today are seen as fairy floss, it was none the less systematic and testable for qualification purposes. In contrast, the practices of the many (although not all) of the UCM modalities mentioned earlier were very often derived from unrecorded 'folk' knowledge passed down verbally from generation to generation. Their lack of scholarly and documentary grounding meant that they, along with the more recently introduced therapies such as homeopathy, chiropractic and osteopathy were mostly rejected in their entirety as fairy floss by the opponents of UCM.

However desirable medical regulation may have seemed in terms of public safety, it was strongly resisted by the followers of UCM because for one thing, the qualifications demanded by Medical Practitioners' Acts set out above were unattainable for its practitioners since their therapies had never been and seemingly could never be included in tertiary medical curricula. That in turn raised the possibility that the failure of UCM practitioners to comply with academic standards would put them outside the law and therefore open to punitive action and even suppression by government.

This point becomes significant in the light of the fact that during the 19th century, as will be detailed in the following chapter, the undisciplined majority in the NSW Lower House rejected repeated attempts to pass medical regulatory legislation. And that majority, as we have seen, was composed mainly of middle and working class people. In other words, the clash between MM and UCM in the late 19th and early 20th centuries in NSW was based on economic and class status as much as it was on medical issues.

It is in the debates of the Lower House detailed that the warlike nature of the contest between MM and UCM can most starkly be seen. The resultant lack of medical regulation meant that medical practice in NSW continued to be a free-for-all in which anyone, as Dr McLaurin pointed out in 1888, could set themselves up as a physician and practice on the bewildered sufferers of 'all the ills known to mankind [sic]'. If a patient died as a result of their treatment by a UCM practitioner, this was considered unexceptionable because at that time of rudimentary medical knowledge, the patients of MM practitioners also suffered a high rate of death at the hands of their tertiary-trained physicians.

CHAPTER 2

The parliamentary theatre

It is against the background outlined in the previous chapter that the 'war' between MM and UCM, as embodied respectively in the Upper and Lower Houses of the NSW Parliament, needs to be seen. One of the chief reasons for the resistance of the Lower House to successive Medical Practitioners' Bills on the surface was not overtly due to a rejection of MM. Instead, the grounds of objection was that they represented attempts to implement 'class legislation', the aim of which was to benefit the medical profession economically. More specifically, in the words of one member, Mr Francis Abigail, the Parliament was being asked to pass a measure 'giving the greatest possible protection to the medical profession'.[1] In May 1880, Mr John Lucas (Canterbury), told the House that he had 'a great objection to class legislation of any description, and he looked upon the Bill as the worst form of class legislation he had ever seen introduced into the House. ... The Bill was a monstrous attempt to protect a few individuals ...'[2]

The views quoted were typical of those held by a majority in the Lower House, which were very often stated with great passion. The wide support for UCM was lamented in an editorial in the *Australasian Medical Gazette*, of March 1883 which stated:

> It should not be forgotten ... that the sympathy both of the average public and more discreditable still, of the authorities, is on the side of quackery. ... there is a well-understood feeling in the public mind - and it extends to all classes - that medical knowledge, like poetry, is

born with the professor, and that quacks are natural geniuses, whom to foster is a duty, and to prosecute is base vindictiveness. [3]

The passion of supporters of UCM is evident from what was said by the member for Northumberland, Mr Ninian Melville, in the 1880 debate in the Lower House on the Medical Practitioners' Bill of that year:

The object of the Bill was stated to be to save suffering humanity from those whom a certain portion of the community were pleased to call quacks. The term 'quack' could only be legitimately applied to a person who pretended to be able to do a certain thing and proved by his action that he was incapable of performing it, and he maintained that if legally qualified men had failed to do what they professed to be able to do they were in every sense quacks as much as persons who were certified to be legally qualified. It was unfortunate that only in a very few cases could the specific result of certain treatment be discovered. If we looked at the prescriptions of the legally qualified men, we should find that they comprised a variety of drugs of such a nature that if the patients for whom they were prescribed knew what they were expected to take they would die from sheer fright.[4]

In that era of pre-scientific medicine and medical practice, Melville's jibe was well-warranted. For instance, it was only in the previous decade that the practice of venesection or bleeding (described in Chapter 1) had finally been abandoned. Pensabene points out that for

... all the major diseases confronting late nineteenth century society - consumption, diphtheria, typhoid, measles, pneumonia and heart disease - the registered doctor had no established cures, nor did he [sic] fully understand the causes of these diseases. [5]

As mentioned above, the 1858 British Medical Practice Act provided a model for medical regulation. Only one year after its passing, Dr Henry Douglass, a member of the NSW Upper House, attempted to have a similar Medical Bill passed. This failed, as did further attempts during the 1860s. Between 1876 and 1900, there were no fewer than 13 separate attempts to have Medical Practitioners' bills passed through the NSW parliament but all failed because, with two exceptions (those of 1886 and 1894-5), they were rejected by the Lower House.

Also responsible for the failure of the Bills was the tendency of the leaders of the Upper House to 'shoot themselves in the foot'. The Bill of 1895 was actually passed by both Houses, but failed to pass into law when the Upper House refused to accept amendments proposed in the Lower House. And when introducing an extensive Medical Practitioners' Bill into the Upper House in August 1897, Sir Arthur Renwick began by giving an assurance, on the basis of his personal contacts, that the British Medical Association 'entirely approve of the provisions of the bill'. He also argued that the findings of the Select Committee into UCM more fully set out below, constituted 'an exposure of the most extraordinary character ... of the prevalence of quackery', and demonstrated the necessity of the legislation. He seems not to have appreciated that both issues were likely to be a 'red-rag-to-a-bull' to the Lower House, as were Bowker's statements that 'a girl was killed and a man was hanged because [a 'quack'] was not prevented from practicing'.[6]

Renwick showed similar lack of perspicacity when he stated that his one reservation about the Bill was its proposals on the constitution of a new Medical Board. The twelve current members he said, felt slighted by the fact that their services would not be automatically continued once the legislation went through. In deference to the sensibilities of these members, whose high status had been recognised by the appointment to the Board in the first place, the House devoted most of the committee stage to trying to devise a complicated formulae to enable the current members to continue in membership, but gradually to be replaced over time.[7]

The record of these deliberations is impressive only in its tedium and of course, in their ultimate futility, because the Lower House refused to consider the Bill. However, one effect of these discussions may have had was to sound a warning that any attempt to reconstitute the Medical Board would be fraught with controversy. Since the introduction of medical regulation had proved to be so highly contentious over so many years, successive NSW governments might have concluded that the introduction of yet another controversial item into the process was something to be avoided if the legislation was ever to be passed. Thus there were no more attempts to change the composition of the Medical Board, which in fact remained unaltered until 1938.

Resistance in the Lower House to successive attempts to pass Medical Practice Bills was not due only to the rejection of what members saw as 'class legislation'. Their hackles were also raised by members of the elite Upper House who saw one of the chief purposes of a Medical Practitioners' Act as being to prohibit the practice of UCM. In the colloquial terms of the day, spokespeople from the MM camp constantly called on government to 'put down quackery'. One of the chief proponents of that view was Dr Richard Bowker, who in his speeches was much given to quoting instances of people being killed by 'quacks' which proved he said, how urgently they needed to be prevented from practicing. He was backed by Dr John Creed mentioned earlier, who was a medical practitioner who had become a full-time politician. As also noted above, he was the editor of the British Medical Association's national journal, *The Australasian Medical Gazette,* in which, as Lloyd points out, 'quackery' was one of the more frequently occurring issues (together with antipathy towards homeopathy).[8]

One reason advanced both at the time and by 20th century writers was that Lower House resistance to the Medical Practitioners' Bills was a result of bribery. This allegation was based on a speech made in the parliament in 1895 by a former Premier Sir George Dibbs, in which he stated that a UCM practitioner, who he refused to name, had not only offered him a bribe to prevent the passage of a Medical Practitioners' Act but boasted that his bribery of other parliamentarians had achieved that purpose on several previous occasions.

This was a serious charge, and as members indignantly pointed out, it impugned the integrity of everyone who voted against the Bill. They challenged Dibbs to call the practitioner to the Bar of the House to answer the allegations. Dibbs never did so. That however, did not prevent his story from being repeated by John Norton, an anti-UCM member of the Lower House who was also the owner of the sensationalist *Truth* newspaper. His speeches in the Parliament tended to reflect its lurid content. He named the practitioner in question as E.H. Botterell, who he said, had done so well out of his 'quackery' that he had 'added house to house and field to field, drove about with a gorgeous equipage, had a beautiful suburban villa and a house on the mountains, station property in the country'. [9]

The bribery charge was repeated by Creed both in the Parliament and in the *Australasian Medical Gazette*, although there, not being protected by parliamentary privilege, he was careful not to mention Botterell's name, referring only to 'a well-known man'. Nor did he make an outright accusation of bribery, stating:

> Of course, I do not venture to connect the expenditure of the money with the failure of the numerous other Medical Bills which passed the Council but failed in another place* to become law, but still it is a subject which readers ... may like to consider in their leisure moments. [10]

That hardly indicates that Creed was sure enough of his facts to challenge Botterell to sue him. In the light of the failure of Dibbs or anyone else to instigate action against Botterell for what after all would have been a blatant attempt to induce impermissible parliamentary behaviour, the charge of bribery seems to have had little substance.

*Parliamentary jargon for the Upper House

Despite their numerous defeats the members of the medical elite in the Upper House relentlessly campaigned to have UCM proscribed. In 1887 Creed convened and chaired a Select Committee appointed by the Upper House 'to inquire into the state and operation of the laws existing for the regulation of the practice of Medicine and Surgery in New South Wales'.[11] That title however, only very partially described the aims of this Select Committee, which were quite transparently an exposure of 'quackery'.

Besides taking evidence from witnesses such as Dr McLaurin (then Chancellor of the University of Sydney) about the uncontrolled state of even orthodox MM, the Select Committee also subpoenaed a good number of UCM practitioners, requiring them to testify about their epistemologies and the administration of their therapies. This was probably designed as a shock tactic because it exposed some outlandish practices and practitioners, apparently in the hope that this would shock the government executive into action.

Among those called was the notorious E.H. Botterell, who proved to be a master of obfuscation. It turned out that his assumption of the title of 'doctor' rested on his having received a diploma from 'Edinburgh University' in Chicago, one of the numerous 'diploma mills' in the USA. Botterell however professed to support a Medical Practitioners' Bill because 'within the last five years Sydney has been inundated with a class of men with no qualifications at all', a good example of his barefaced effrontery, given that he had no genuine qualifications either. It also demonstrated that when it came to eliminating economic competition, he was as pro-regulation as any member of the medical elite.

Among others examined was a herbalist, one Michael Green, whose medical epistemology may be judged by the following exchange with the Creed:

Q. When did you study medicine?

A. About twenty-five years ago.

Q. Under whom?

A. My own; as it came into my head.

Q. You never had any teachers?

A. No; only the Almighty ....The Bible I study is my
   guide to botany, and Almighty God is my physician,
   my teacher, and my guide in every shape and form.

Some evidence of a homeopathic practitioner, William Moore,
was considered so obscene that it was deleted from the record of
the committee. However, in 1886 Creed had referred extensively
to Moore in a speech to the Upper House. After noting that there
were no ladies present (he seems to have ignored the fact that
'ladies' could and did read the Parliamentary Hansard), Creed
quoted from a pamphlet published by Moore in which he claimed
he could provide a means by which men could protect themselves
from being 'copper-blown' by a woman who, during sexual
intercourse, held a deep breath 'while the semen is passing from
the male; wind from the female has been known in many instance
to pass under these circumstances, into the male, and to inflate him
like a bladder'.

For the supporters of UCM medicine as well as for government
politicians, the hilarity and shock effect of such anecdotes was
probably counteracted by Creed's statement that while Moore had
a large practice, 'I think I must have convinced hon. members that
he is so grossly ignorant that he should not be allowed to practice
at all.' [12]

As related earlier, one of Creed's particular targets were
practitioners of homeopathy, who also figured prominently among
the 'quacks' summoned by his Select Committee in the following
year. Although in its report the committee stated: 'We are not
prepared to recommend that any person should be prohibited

from practicing medicine…' and Creed himself repeated this in the parliament, there appears to have been some ambivalence in his position. While himself giving evidence to the Select Committee, he was asked: 'Do you think that disease would be more under control if there were no unauthorised practitioners who did not understand their business'. He simply replied 'Yes'. And while his committee may not have called for the banning of UCM, it did recommend that all UCM practitioners be legislatively forced to add the words 'Unregistered by the Medical Board' to their advertisements and also to display them on plates 'in some conspicuous place open to public view'.[11]

This recommendation was never implemented and in fact the strenuous attempts by the proponents of MM to impose controls on UCM were probably counter-productive and actually delayed the introduction of full medical regulation. The *Australasian Medical Gazette* lamented in an editorial of February 1898 that while the Select Committee had exposed 'the danger to the public and the urgent necessity for legislation', it was 'almost impossible to realize that no action was taken, the then Premier, Sir Henry Parkes, quietly ignoring it'.[13]

That was just one example of the ways in which the medical elite proved incapable of bringing successive governments in NSW 'on side' in the four decades between 1860 and 1900. The continuing hostility of these MPs to UCM and the insistence by some on the need for governments to 'put down quackery', in all likelihood merely succeeded in increasing the intransigent resistance of the Lower House to the introduction of medical regulation. And being an elected body, the Lower House undoubtedly, although composed entirely of men, reflected the support of UCM by the majority of the population of NSW.

CHAPTER 3

Infamous sleight of hand

Its lack of medical regulation left NSW, the most populous and economically advanced of the Australian colonies, looking increasingly isolated and idiosyncratic. Not that the NSW governmental interest and activity in health care had lagged behind the other Australian jurisdictions. While the 1856 *Journal of the Legislative Council* carried only two reports relating to health issues, these being those of the Medical Adviser to government (who was exclusively concerned with vaccination activities) and that of the Health Officer (who likewise was exclusively concerned with quarantine issues),[1] the rapidly increasing population forced the change noted by Davis when he recorded that: 'The second half of the century was marked by increasing State interest and support for medical activity both private and public, curative and preventative.' [2]

Thus in 1886 the *Journal of the Legislative Council* carried reports about a large number of 'charitable institutions', i.e. government subsidised hospitals, including four in Sydney and 68 in country areas as well as eight government asylums for the 'infirm and destitute'. Besides the 131 vaccinators reported to be active in that 1887, there were also 96 medical officers serving in institutions such as jails, asylums and special schools as well as in country towns.[3] By 1900 the number of hospitals had risen to 121.[4]

This increasing governmental involvement in health matters was based solely on MM as was the growing health bureaucracy. And that the health bureaucrats were as anti-UCM as any of the parliamentarians in the Upper House is evident from a report to the Legislative Council submitted by Dr Anderson Stuart, Medical Advisor to the Government, in 1894, in which he stated:

> The question has arisen during the year as to whether unqualified medical practitioners should be appointed to medical officerships of subsidised hospitals; and it has been decided that in no case shall a hospital subsidised by Government employ either as a paid or an honorary medical officer any person who is not a legally qualified medical practitioner according to the law of New South Wales [5]

At the time there was no such law in NSW, but this major policy decision, taken without any reference to the Parliament, obviously excluded any UCM practitioners from the governmental health system.

However, a major problem with that policy was that without any medical regulatory law in NSW, it was impossible to know who was entitled to be recognised as a legally qualified medical practitioner. While the health bureaucracy were no doubt aware of this, it must have been obvious that there was no hope of getting any medical legislation through the Parliament if it originated in the Upper House or was associated with its anti-UCM medical elite in any way.

At that stage the government must have been desperate to have a Medical Practitioners' Act in the statute books. Elementary medical regulatory legislation had been passed in Tasmania as far back as 1838, in Victoria in 1862[6], in New Zealand in 1866,[7] in South Australia in 1880[8], in Queensland in 1867[9] and in Western Australia in 1894[10]. Similar medical regulation was also advancing apace in the United States, where according to Starr, every State had passed the necessary legislation by 1901.[11]

Thus the NSW government devised a strategy which between

1898 and 1901 resulted in not one, but three Medical Practitioners' Acts being passed. Two of these were testimony to the political power of UCM because obviously the government was being forced to apply a Machiavellian strategy when it finagled the first, the Medical Practitioners' Act (No. 26) of 1898 into law. Despite its title, this Act almost exactly duplicated the Medical Witnesses Acts of 1838 and its amendment Act of 1855, merely specifying the qualifications required of physicians called to give evidence at coronial inquests.

There were no debates on this Act, which was passed through all its stages in one fell swoop in the Lower House in July 1898 along with a long list of other 'consolidation' Acts.[12] However curious this Act may have seemed – and still seems today – its title signalled the government's determination to get a Medical Practitioner's Act onto the statute book no matter in what form and this was the first step in that direction.

The second step was taken two years later when the Medical Practitioners' Amendment Act (No 33, 1900) was introduced into the Parliament. The way it was handled again evidences a careful strategy designed not to alarm supporters and practitioners of UCM. Firstly, the legislation originated in the Lower, not the Upper House; secondly it was piloted through that House by a member who had no connections with the medical elite and thirdly the Bill was drafted in a minimalist fashion, containing only three working clauses.

The first made it an offence for any unqualified person to assume 'the name or title of a physician, doctor of medicine, or surgeon... or description implying that he is legally qualified'. The penalty was severe: a fine of £50 and £5 for each day during which the offence was committed or alternatively a jail term of 12 months. However, there was nothing in the Act forbidding anyone without the specified qualifications from practising in the medical field; anyone was free to do so provided they did not call themselves a doctor, surgeon or legally qualified person.

That could hardly be construed as an attempt to 'put down quackery' and given their lack of objections to this Act, it seems the 'quacks' themselves did not see it that way. Perhaps that was because giving themselves the title of 'doctor' might at the time have been a kiss-of-death for any UCM practitioner working in a population in which so many people were hostile to the medical profession.

The member who piloted the Bill through the Lower House was R.A. Price who, while he was a supporter of MM, could be seen as an 'honest, working man'. His chief argument was that no one would ever justify a workman (sic) claiming trade qualifications which he did not possess.[13] It was not a debating point which would have occurred to anyone in the medical elite. That after rejecting Medical Practice Bills over the previous forty years, the Lower House allowed this one through with practically no debate, indicates that a deal had been stitched up beforehand behind closed doors with the supporters of UCM in the House. They had very likely agreed to pass the Bill on condition that it did not interfere with the practice of UCM in any way.

Predictably, the Bill also sailed through the Upper House without any opposition and one significant change in what was now an Act, was the insertion of the word 'Registration' into the name of the Medical Board. That signalled that those physicians whose names appeared on the Medical Register were now not merely qualified to give evidence in the Coronial Court, but were legally entitled to practice medicine in the State. That was something the medical profession in NSW had been striving for the previous four decades of the 19th century and that passage of time through both the 20th and 21st centuries has not in any way diminished the desirability of the status not only for doctors but also for any one practising any kind of healing modality, including UCM.

Yet while the 1901 Act would have pleased the government and bureaucracy, it was far less pleasing to the medical elite. That was because the only standards-maintenance mechanism it contained was the power it gave to the Medical Board to de-register any doctor who had been convicted of a crime in a court of law. In contrast, what the elite wanted was for the Act to include the same disciplinary instrument as that included in the original British Medical Practice Act of 1858, which gave the General Medical Council exclusive power to deregister any practitioner it adjudged to have been guilty of 'infamous conduct in any professional respect'.

What was infamous conduct? The medical profession replied in effect, that this was a 'priestly mystery' which only they understood. This archaic and obscure wording was in fact the same as that contained in the statutes adopted by the Royal College of Physicians when it was founded in the 16th century. And that wording Berlant points out, 'did not include mistakes or incompetence' short of gross malpractice and gross incompetence.[14] In other words, infamous conduct related only to behaviour, particularly public drunkenness or addiction to drugs, adjudged likely to bring the medical profession into disrepute. It did not cover poor or injurious medical practice. However far-fetched that position seems, it was upheld by the British High Court in what became the famous 'Allinson case' of 1894. The Allinson referred to was a medical practitioner who had been deregistered by the General Medical Council (GMC) for publishing advertisements in which he disparagingly compared his own curative record with that of his fellow medical practitioners. His appeal against the GMC's action was dismissed by the High Court and in his judgement which set a long-standing precedent, Lord Justice Lopes provided the following definition of infamous conduct:

> If a medical man in the pursuit of his profession has done something ... which will be reasonably regarded as disgraceful or dishonourable by his professional brethren of good repute and competency, then it is open to the General Medical Council, if that be shown, to say that he has been guilty of infamous conduct in a professional respect. (p763).

In that judgement, Lopes was in fact affirming that only the medical profession could pronounce on what constituted 'infamous conduct,' which in fact meant that the judgements of the profession as expressed through bodies such as the GMC and the Medical Board in NSW, fell outside the jurisdiction of the courts. In other words, the Lopes judgement affirmed and entrenched the institutional autonomy of medicine which indicates that among the upper classes in Britain and therefore in its overseas possessions such as New South Wales, the ancient profession of medicine enjoyed if not a semi-divine then an extremely exalted status.

For the medical elite in NSW, the failure of the 1900 Medical Practitioners' Act Amendment Act described above to include the 'infamous conduct' provision was a major flaw and under the leadership of Creed, they set about remedying it. Creed was an experienced parliamentarian and thus without the knowledge of the government, he drafted another Act containing the 'infamous conduct' clause which gave the Medical Board the sole competence to enforce it. His Act was introduced into the Lower House at 10 p.m. in early December 1900 when attendance was low. Creed was no doubt gratified when the Bill passed through all its stages - first, second, third readings plus the committee stage - in 11 minutes.[15]

It was speedily then sent to the Upper House, but here it encountered unexpected obstacles. The first was thrown up by the leader of the House Sir Frank Suttor, who protested that having passed the earlier Medical Practitioners' Amendment Act, the House was being asked to pass it for a second time. Creed was able to bluster his way past this obstacle, only to be confronted by another more serious one in the person of Dr John Nash, who being based in the Newcastle area, was not numbered among the Sydney medical elite. Referring to the Allinson case, he noted that the 'infamous conduct' clause had caused a great deal of difficulty in Britain and asked Creed for a definition of the term. Creed's reply was: 'It is impossible to define it'.[16] Nobody questioned whether an indefinable concept could or should be read into law.

Creed was not alone in defending the clause, particularly because Nash's objection had caused near-panic not only among the medical elite, but also other members of the House who wanted to see the legislation passed. One such was Dr William Cullen (he was a doctor of laws, not a medical doctor) who declared:

> I think we ought to take what the gods send us, and be thankful. We have been trying to legislate in this direction for a very long time, and now, when we find two bills passed through the Assembly in one week each giving us an instalment of what has long been desired by the people, I think we ought to pass it.[15]

In the end Nash agreed to drop his objections and the Bill was read into law as the Medical Practitioner's Further Amendment Act (No 70, 1900). Its passing did not mean the repeal of the previous two Acts, but while they remained in force, Creed's Act with its 'infamous conduct' clause became the chief instrument of medical discipline. The validity of that clause was resoundingly confirmed by the Supreme Court of NSW in 1917 when it upheld the Medical Board's deregistration of a doctor for infamous conduct, stating that 'this court is very loath to disturb the finding of a Board of professional men whose knowledge of what may be termed professional misconduct must be very much greater than the Court can possess.'[17]

The passing of the three Medical Practitioner Acts between 1898 and 1900 set out what was to become the legal groundwork for the standing of MM over against that UCM throughout the 20th and into the 21st century, in terms of which, while UCM was allowed to exist and indeed flourish, MM was recognised by the government as the 'official' medical epistemology in the Colony/State. As such these Acts, which were consolidated into one Act in 1912, immensely strengthened the position of the medical profession and therefore of MM in NSW. And that would have far-reaching effects on MM's battles with UCM later in the 20th century.

CHAPTER 4

The end of UCM's political road

It was federation or nothing. When in the last years of the 19th century the bickering, mutually suspicious Australian colonies agreed to join themselves together in the Commonwealth of Australia, it was on condition that, following the American model of federalism, they be constitutionally empowered to retain sovereign control over important aspects of their governance, health being one of these. Thus while on January 1, 1901, the Commonwealth Parliament came into existence, it was mainly concerned with national issues such as foreign affairs and defence. For its part, the New South Wales Parliament, without missing a beat, continued to meet and legislate as it had done ever since 1856.

If the proceedings of that Parliament are anything to go by, all was quiet on the MM/UCM battle front for close on 40 years after the passing of the three Medical Practitioners' Acts in 1900/1901. However, while the noisy 19th century confrontations between the protagonists of MM and UCM were no longer heard in Parliamentary debates, there were continuous and important developments in the health field which favoured MM. Governmental realisation of the importance of health issues was signaled by the creation of the State's first Department of Health with its own Minister in 1913. While at that time the staff amounted to a little over 100[1], by 1938 that number had grown to close on 1,400 working in 25 sub-divisions[2].

In the lack of scientific surveys, it is impossible to gauge the effect of these developments on the practice and following of UCM during these decades. However, one reflection of its continuing widespread usage were the plentiful advertisements placed by its practitioners in the print media of the time. Obviously if these had not produced results in the form of a steady stream of customers, the advertisements would have disappeared in time. They did not disappear.

On the basis of its growing scientific understandings and therapeutic efficacy, MM was riding ever higher both in public esteem and in governmental recognition. Still, one major reason for continuing MM dis-satisfaction was the lack of an adequate Medical Practitioners' Act. Although the three Acts of 1901 Acts had been consolidated in 1912, this new Act was still a very brief instrument containing only 12 clauses, which besides laying down the qualifications required of medical practitioners and the notorious 'infamous conduct' clause, did little more than specify the size and composition of the Medical Board. This Act became increasingly unfit for its purpose since not only did the population continue to increase rapidly, rising from 1,777,534 in 1912 to 2,735,695 in 1938 (35%), but the number of medical practitioners in the State expanded even more quickly from 3,213 in 1912 to 6,035 (53%) in 1938[3]. Making the minimalist 1912 Act increasingly anomalous was that other health occupations including pharmacy,[4] dentistry[5], nursing[6] and optometry[7] had been regulated by legislation far more comprehensive than the 1912 Medical Practitioners' Act.

While there is evidence of a consciousness in government that that badly needed to be expanded and updated, the 19th century struggles set out in the previous chapters had left a long institutional memory which seems to have discouraged any attempts to pass another Act. This can be deduced from an anecdote told by Herbert FitzSimons who was Minister of Health in 1930s. In the later stages of his long parliamentary career, he related in the Upper House:

> I well recall that in 1936 I first discussed proposals for the new Medical practitioners Act with the Crown Solicitor, Mr Clarke, and the Parliamentary Draftsman,

Mr. McCrae. I remember Mr. Clarke looking at me quizzically in my office in the Department of Health and saying: 'Are you really serious about attempting a new Medical Practitioners Act?' I said, 'Yes, Cabinet has directed it.' He said: 'I shall just tell you this. In the department somewhere there are probably the remains of twenty six previous drafts of Medical Practitioners Acts, some of which were taken only to the rough draft stage, some of which were printed and some of which were actually introduced, but as far as I know none ever succeeded in getting approval'[8].

What the sceptical the 'Sir Humphrey' of his day failed to take into account was the radical change in the functioning of the NSW parliament over the past half-century. From the 1890s onwards, the Labor Electoral League, forerunner of the Australian Labor Party which was founded in 1908, not only dramatically increased its representation, but insisted that anyone elected on its ticket take 'The Pledge' to vote with the Party on every issue, on pain of expulsion if they failed to do so.[9] As described in Chapter 2, this 'party discipline' (which was nothing new, having long been the rule in the British Parliament[10]) guaranteed that all legislation introduced by Labor governments would be passed. That proved so effective that it was speedily adopted by Labor's opponents who also formed themselves into organised political parties.

Herbert Fitzsimons, a tough ex-army officer, was a member of one such party, the United Australia Party (forerunner of today's Liberal Party) which appointed him Minister for Health after it came to power in 1932. After they were re-elected in 1935, he and his party, as can be seen from the quotation above, resolved to pass a full-blown, up-to-date Medical Practitioners' Act and began cautious moves in that direction in following year. The final steps were not taken until their third election victory in early 1938 cleared the way for FitzSimons to introduce the most extensive and sophisticated medical regulatory legislation n NSW to that date. With seven sections and 53 clauses covering a wide range of issues pertaining to the regulation of the medical profession and medical practice, the new Act ensured that NSW would at last come into line with other Australian States and overseas jurisdictions.

It might also be remarked in passing that this Act enormously strengthened the position of the medical profession. Not only did it extend and tighten the provisions relating to the admission of candidates to the profession, it also laid down that only registered practitioners were permitted to hold appointments, honorary or non-honorary, as medical officers in public hospitals , to sign death certificates or to sign any legal certificates. Although these stipulations, as we have seen earlier, had been applied since 1894 in terms of health departmental policy, this was the first time they had been given the force of law, something that constituted a major reinforcement of MM's dominance.

When he introduced the 1938 legislation, Fitzsimons said its aims could be summed up as greater control of the medical profession, control of the manufacturers of patent medicine and control of 'lay practitioners'. The 'lay practitioners' were the proponent s of UCM and this was the first move against them in the 20th century. However the 'control' shrewdly did not inhibit their freedom to practise but simply prohibited them from advertising. On the face of things, this was perfectly justifiable; doctors after all, had always been prohibited from advertising by their professional ethics and that UCM practitioners were free to advertise seemingly created a very un-level playing field.

However not being able to advertise threatened to deprive UCM practitioners of much of their commercial oxygen and not surprisingly, this stipulation provoked an enormous furore in the Parliament which demonstrated that the fervor of the proponents of UCM had by no means diminished compared to that of their 19th century political forebears. Their strength of feeling is evident in the way they took the almost unheard of step of opposing the first reading of the Bill and of course fiercely re-iterated their opposition during the Bill's second reading. On this score, the

NSW Parliament differed sharply from Victoria where, according to Pensabene, remarks favourable to MM made in its parliament in the 1930s showed that: 'Gone was the old hostility shown to the medical practitioner in the previous century'.[11]

In NSW, very little other than the 'old hostility' was in evidence in the Lower House. During the first reading debate the member for Bathurst, Christopher Kelly, told the House that ever since the Bill had been mooted, he had received 'quite a sheaf of letters from people who ... generally point out the value of the lay practitioner and what wonderful, and in some cases, miraculous cures have been performed. One gentleman wrote to me the other day and said he had no faith in doctors at all. It may be an open question as to whether they are any better than the lay practitioner'. To illustrate that, his correspondent recounted an anecdote in which he told of how his wife, he himself and the doctor on a ship on which they were travelling, had all come down with the 'flu. The ship's captain had given the writer a bottle of rum as a remedy and having drunk the rum,

> I sent for the doctor for my wife. The doctor prescribed a certain medicine, the prescription being written in Latin. Then the doctor told me he himself had influenza. I asked him what he was taking himself and he said he was just drinking water and plenty of it. I drank the rum, my wife took the doctor's medicine and the doctor drank water and we all got better around the same time.

More serious evidence of continuing scepticism about the claims of MM is evident in a statement by James Heffron, (later to become leader of the NSW Labor Party and Premier of the State) who told the House that the medical profession had always been extremely conservative and that its members had consistently resisted the discoveries of laymen. This theme of the conservatism of MM over against the 'cutting edge' innovatory nature of UCM medicine was taken up again and again by speakers in both the first and second reading debates on the bill. In the words of James Arkins, a member of the United Australia Party, 'As one delves into the history of medicine, one finds that generally the discoveries have been made by the unorthodox medical man'. The names of Jenner, Lister, Pasteur and Simpson (the inventor of chloroform) were all mentioned as being among those whose discoveries had been initially scorned by the medical profession.

It was not only MM in general but the NSW branch of the British Medical Association (BMA) which was a particular target of attack since it was seen to be the *eminence grise* behind the Bill. Arthur Tonge charged that 'this was not a doctor's bill, it was a BMA bill'. In debates in the Upper House, the BMA was described as 'the greatest union that Australia possesses' by one speaker. So fierce were the accusations against the BMA that it felt constrained to deny them in an editorial in the *Medical Journal of Australia* [12] which the Minister also felt constrained to quote in Parliament to support his assertion that 'any suggestion … that this bill is the product of the British Medical Association is without foundation, and untrue' [13].

Had the situation in the Lower House been the same as it was in the later 19th century, no doubt this Bill would have been blocked by its opponents by means of filibusters or by ensuring that there was no quorum present or simply ignoring it and letting it lapse. In 1938 however, the Australian Labor Party which ever since it was formed in NSW in 1908 had been the chief standard bearer of the UCM cause, was hopelessly split between two separate parties each claiming to be the true bearers of the Labor brand, one led by James Heffron, the other by the ex-NSW Premier Jack Lang.

In any in case, being in opposition, the two Labor Parties constituted a minority of MPs in the House and therefore were in no position to block the Bill. What made its passing even more certain was that the leaders of Fitzsimmons's Australia United Party could now invoke party discipline. One of the most telling illustrations of the effect of party discipline is that James Arkins quoted above, one of the most bitter critics of the Bill, none the less consistently voted for it. The reason could be that, having been elected as a Labor representative in 1915, moving into the National Party twelve years later finally into the ruling United Australia Party[14], he had become a professional politician, reliant on his parliamentary income and therefore needing to hold his seat. As his statements quoted above make clear, he was still a fervent proponent of UCM and in party room discussions behind closed doors he probably fiercely attacked the proposed Act and vowed to continue his attacks in open debate in the Parliament. But while Fitzsimons and other party leaders were willing to tolerate that, he would also have known that voting against the Bill would in terms of party discipline call down a parliamentary death sentence on his head.

Even though there was practically no support for the Bill among speakers during the debates in the Lower House, where it was criticised even by members of the government, the Bill was passed on party lines in August 1938.[13] Then, in line with the situation of the 19th century when Medical Practitioners' bills were invariably passed by the Upper House, the Bill had a much smoother passage through that Chamber, finding plentiful support from the floor. Here the second reading debate was completed in one day without a division.[16]

When this new Medical Practitioners' Act was assented to in December 1938, that signaled a final end to the political dominance of UCM which had lasted in the NSW Parliament ever since it was granted responsible government in 1856. But it was not only party discipline which brought this about; notably lacking in the arguments advanced by UCM proponents in the 1938 debates, were any of the class-based critiques of the medical profession which had figured so largely in the previous century. Moreover, that there was no visible popular movement outside of the Parliament supporting the political resistance to the new Act, indicated that in the face of MM advances in medical science and its exclusive recognition by government, middle and working-class support for UCM if it had not vanished altogether, was much diminished. Although the newspapers of the time gave extensive coverage to the Parliamentary debates and to the issue itself, they tended to maintain a neutral editorial position. Deprived of its Parliamentary platform and also of its ability to bring itself to public notice through advertising , UCM suffered a long eclipse in NSW.

CHAPTER 5

The dominance and decline of Mainstream Medicine 1938-1987

The 1938 Medical Practitioner's Act seemed to signal that Mainstream Medicine (MM) had won its 'war' with UnConventional Medicine (UCM) in New South Wales and was ready to dominate the health field in that State from a position of supreme, unquestioned authority. For the greater part of the half century after 1938, MM was the only medical modality recognised by governments and was used by a growing majority of the community. It was also the only modality to which the media paid any attention and it alone was taught in the academic sphere. As a result, for the next four decades, the extensive array of UCM therapies set out in Chapter 1 largely became invisible in the public domain.

UCM's apparent decline aided MM's ascent to a peak of power resulting from the increasing understanding by both its researchers and practitioners of the microbial and viral causes of infectious disease, as well as discoveries of how these could be treated and cured. These advances were the result of scientific research carried out among others by medical pioneers such as Pasteur, Koch and Yersin in the 19th and early 20th centuries. At the same time the development of anaesthesia and the work of figures such as Joseph Lister made surgery much safer and more successful and therefore ever more widely practised.

These advances led to a paradigm shift in the practice of MM which saw the final discarding of the ancient humoral approaches set out in Chapter 1. From the later 19th century onwards, MM became increasingly characterised as *scientific medicine,* the research efforts and methodologies of which produced the 'miracle cures' effected by sulfonimides and streptomycin during the first half of the 20th century. And of course, most notably, was the epochal discovery of penicillin and other antibiotics. Spurred into mass production by WWII from 1943 onwards, these made formerly fatal diseases such as pneumonia routinely and quickly curable while at the same time making it possible to altogether eliminate formely killer diseases such as smallpox.

These advances in the understanding and treatment of disease 'strengthened a growing sense that biomedicine was bringing humanity to a promised land of vibrant health and freedom from disease.'[1] Armed with new 'wonder drugs', as well as the success of mass immunisation programs, MM was finally able to negate Ninian Melville's 1880 Parliamentary jibe that its frequent failure to effect the cures it promised, made it as 'quackish' as UCM.

The Buledelah loggers

Yet while its therapeutic advances resulted in ever more acceptance by and growing admiration for MM among the general population, there was one blot on its reputation which was to have significant sociological effects on its standing. That was the way its practitioners, its institutions and also governments dealt with inevitable therapeutic failures and harms that patients suffered while undergoing treatments at the hands of MM practitioners and institutions. In other words, one of the most significant challenges to the dominance of MM in the mid- to late 20th century was the question of patient complaints. The almost total lack of redress for aggrieved patients during that period was reflected in the case related by John Hawkins, a Labor MP, in evidence he provided in the lead-up to the passing of the Medical Practitioners Act of 1938.

Hawkins related how the negligence of a doctor in the village hospital of Buladelah, about 150km north of Sydney, directly contributed to the death of an injured 19-year-old worker in a forestry camp in the district. When the man fell seriously ill after a workplace accident, his workmates carried him 4km over bush tracks on an improvised stretcher to the hospital in Buledelah. There the crusty old doctor on duty truculently asked who would pay for the costs of his treatment. ('Free' hospital cover did not come into Australia until long after this.)

After the workmates said they would cover all costs and urged that the man needed to be taken to Newcastle hospital, the doctor demanded who would pay for the phone call to summon an ambulance. Again the loggers said they would pay, but after they left the hospital, the doctor did nothing more than examine the man and diagnose blood poisoning, leaving him in a bed outside on a veranda for the rest of the night and next day without treatment. When his workmates visited him the following evening, they found him semi-comatose, but when they protested to the doctor, he ordered them out of the hospital. Although the young man was eventually taken by ambulance to Newcastle hospital, he died there.

So outraged were the workmates that, no doubt donning jackets and ties, they took their complaint to Hawkins as their local MP. He in turn took the case to Minister for Health Herbert Fitzsimmons, who however claimed that under the current Medical Practitioners' Act (that passed in 1912), he had no power to act against the doctor. In fact he did have such a power in terms of that Act; the old doctor could surely have been charged with 'infamous conduct in professional respect'. But very likely the Minister would only have invoked that clause had the doctor been drunk or under the influence of drugs while on duty, which would have been considered a much more heinous offence than allowing a man to die through bloody-minded negligence. The best the Minister could think of was to refer the case to the Medical Association , but since the doctor was not a member of that organisation, it had no grounds for taking action.

Thus the loggers were helpless to do anything more; obviously they never thought of taking the case to the media because their tale of sacrificial mateship was never reported anywhere and is recorded only in the NSW parliamentary Hansard.[2] Still, because of their long-term deleterious effects on the standing of MM, cases such as this were to have an indirect but important effect on the course of its war with UCM.

The Windsor Hospital incident – springboard to power

Although the way MM's domination was exercised on a national level, particularly through the Australian Medical Association, has been well chronicled[3-6], moving the focus to NSW highlights some of the political factors which swept MM to unprecedented heights of power and influence during the mid-20th century. One of the most prominent examples of this development in NSW was the outcome of an incident which began in late 1961 when a Dr J.F. Boag, a Visiting Medical Officer working in the Windsor District Hospital about 100km west of Sydney, was seeing private patients in his surgery at the time he was supposed to be on duty at the hospital.

When a six-year old boy with an arm fractured in two places by a fall from a horse was brought into the hospital for treatment, Boag directed that the boy be brought to his surgery. When that was done and the boy's fractures were attended to, Boag demanded a fee of £10 (equivalent to around $100 in today's terms). Had the treatment been undertaken at the hospital, it would have been free.

That story too, was initially unnoticed by the media, but it was considered serious enough for the Windsor Hospital Board to ask Boag to attend an inquiry on December 18, 1961. When he refused, claiming he had not been given enough notice, he was suspended from his Visiting Medical Officer position. In reaction, all the other nine Visiting Medical Officers withdrew their services from the hospital. That had a dire consequence when a man died because there was no doctor to treat him at the hospital.

This time the case was reported to a newspaper, the *Sydney Morning Herald* , which on December 26, printed the story under a large headline: 'NO DOCTOR AVAILABLE. MAN DIES'. The man, having been injured in a water skiing accident on the Hawkesbury River, had been taken by his friends by car to the Windsor Hospital. There, with no doctors on duty due to the Visiting Medical Officers' strike, they were directed to the surgery of one of the strikers, but could get no response when they knocked on the door (it was a Sunday). They then drove the injured man to Parramatta hospital, but he died on the way.

The story caused a great public outcry so much so that, after being contacted by the Hospitals Commission (the body which at the time had oversight of all hospitals in the State), the Visiting Medical Officers agreed that while on strike, they would treat emergency cases at the hospital.

The following day the *Herald* again carried a major article under the headline 'Doctor Dispute: Sheahan Sees Need for Ethics Review' (Sheahan being the Minister for Health at the time). It also ran an editorial entitled 'The Duty of Doctors' in which it attacked the striking Visiting Medical Officers for their 'false sense of loyalty to a colleague'. The editorial stated:

> Such an extreme decision by a group of doctors virtually to boycott their own hospital is rare, if not unprecedented, in the annals of the medical profession. But the fact that it could occur at all, points to a lowering of former professional standards. Many complaints received by the Department of Health... show that there is a more extensive withholding of services and relaxation of diligence than this extreme case would suggest.

The *Herald* and other newspapers for days on end ran major stories on the incident and the subsequent four-day long inquiry by the Hospital Board in January, 1962. On January 11, the main front-page headline of the *Herald* read: 'Board Dismisses Doctor: New

Angry Clashes at Inquiry' while Boag's dismissal was described as a 'Hitler regime tactic' by his counsel, Clive Evatt QC.

Confrontations of this kind made excellent news material for all media and the resultant press coverage made it imperative for government to be seen to be acting to ensure that the Windsor Hospital debacle was not repeated. Labor Minister Sheahan, mentioned earlier, thus set about a major revision of the 1938 Medical Practitioners' Act. He proceeded carefully, his first move being to call the 'ethics conference' alluded to by the *Herald* headline quoted above, on January 23, 1962. It was attended by representatives from his Health Department, the Medical Board, the Australian Medical Association (AMA - it had changed its name from the British Medical Association) and also a lecturer in medical ethics from the University of Sydney.

The conference appears to have been a stormy one. Health Minister Sheahan later told the Parliament that there had been a 'frank' discussion and 'differences of opinion', [7] a typical parliamentary euphemism for a blazing row. Although he did not specify the main points of difference, the medical representatives were probably reacting against his proposition that the definition of 'infamous conduct' should be extended to include refusal by a doctor to see patients in an emergency. Despite the objections, just such a clause was incorporated into the amended Act. This was the first time that there had been any specification or definition of 'infamous conduct' in NSW legislation.

Still, if the 1963 Act was designed to rein in the medical profession, it had exactly the opposite effect. One reason was that during the uproar about the Windsor Hospital incident, it emerged that disgruntled patients were directing complaints about sub-standard healthcare by both doctors and hospitals to the office of the Minister Sheahan. At the January conference mentioned above, Sheahan had expressed concern about 'the number of complaints being made against the Department of Health in regard to the failure on the part of members of the profession to answer what were said to be emergency calls'. He objected to this addition to his workload and that of his Department and, to judge by the legislation he had drafted, was intent on discouraging the flow of health complaints, siding with the medical profession against complainants.

This was a period when the Labor Party (which had been in power in NSW since 1941), in the person of Minister Sheahan anyway, seemingly softened and very nearly reversed its traditional hostility to the AMA. Thus not only was the 'infamous conduct' clause adopted without question in the 1963 Act, but Minister Sheahan went out of his way to defend it, declaring : 'Nobody can attempt to define infamous conduct. To try to do so would be like Mr Speaker, trying to define improper conduct in this House'.[7] It was a not a good analogy; the Standing Orders of Parliament define improper conduct very closely (e.g. loud and persistent interjections) and there are a range of prescribed penalties for such conduct: loud and persistent interjectors may be suspended or ejected from the House. No one, even in Sheahan's own Labor Party, made any attempt to point this out.

Their failure to question or contradict Sheahan on this point, let alone vote against it, indicates that the socially-exalted status the profession had enjoyed ever since the passing of the Medical Practice Act of 1901, was still largely unquestioned sixty years later. The continued incorporation of 'infamous conduct' as the chief ground for medical discipline in the 1963 Act was, as will be demonstrated, one of the most important pillars of MM dominance and constituted a visible manifestation of the peak of power it attained in the mid-20th century. And it was paradoxical that it was the Labor Party, the longstanding critic of the medical profession, which was responsible for exalting the profession to that peak.

The rising tide of patient complaints

What the case of the Buledelah loggers indicated was the almost complete lack of any idea of patient rights in NSW for most of the 20th century. But in fact this lack had originally been reflected in the elementary Medical Practitioner's Acts of 1901 and 1912, which gave no recognition to the existence of patient complaints, let alone specifying how these might be dealt with.

Not until 1938 was the issue of patient complaints recognised in the extensive Medical Practitioners' Act of that year. Yet while up to then the only channel for registering and seeking redress for complaints lay through the courts, the number of such complaints was growing as the 20th century progressed. Thus, whereas in the 25 years between 1912 and 1938 the number of disciplinary charges against medical practitioners based on patient complaints was only 12, in April 1940 the Medical Registration Board reported that in that year alone, disciplinary charges were pending against eight medical practitioners.[8]

That report was made in terms of the mechanisms for dealing with patient complaints set up by the 1938 Medical Practitioner's Act, which had specified that these should be channelled to a newly constituted Medical Tribunal by the State's Board of Health. That Board of Health, originally set up in 1881 to deal with the outbreak of epidemics, consisted of both medical and and non-medical members, the latter in the majority. It had no full-time officials and only met monthly. The choice of this unlikely body to handle health complaints was possibly because no one could think of anything else at the time. But that it was given this new duty indicated a growing awareness of health complaints, the Board being tasked with referring any complaints it thought deserving of disciplinary action to the newly constituted Medical Tribunal mentioned above, which was in fact simply the Medical Registration Board presided over by a District Court judge.

Although the Board of Health did not prove to be particularly sympathetic to individual complainants, none the less the number of disciplinary cases it sent to the Tribunal began increasing, especially in the late 1950s and early 1960s.[9] But because the system set up by the 1938 Act proved to be both clumsy and ineffectual, complainants were increasingly using unofficial channels for their grievances, chief among which were newspapers .

That the use of this non-official channel was a cause of concern to the medical profession was evidenced by the establishment in September 1956 by the NSW branch of the Australian Medical Association of a Public Relations Committee. The main aim of this Committee was to counter the negative attitudes of the Press to the medical profession. The sense of concern evidenced by the formation of the Publc Relations Committee was, on the face of things, somewhat surprising. While the ever-increasing technical expertise and therapeutic successes of MM called forth media praise, what was concerning for the Australian Medical Association (the AMA from this point onwards) during this period, was that newspapers were also more than willing to carry strong critiques of the medical profession. Examples of such continuing critiques, considered at a Public Relations Committee meeting in June 1962, included an editorial in the *Sun Herald* in which doctors were accused of carelessness and incompetence with headlines such as 'The scandal of American doctors', (*Sun Herald* 7/6/1962) and 'Medicine men talk gibberish' (*Sunday Mirror* 10/6/1962).

In his response to articles and headlines such as these, the AMA's Director of Communications prepared a submission which is worth quoting at length because it so well encapsulates reasons for the problematic public image of the AMA and the medical profession as a whole.

> The Association has very friendly relations with the press [but the press] finds much more 'news value' in criticism of the medical profession than in the Association's replies. Whenever strong criticisms are made they usually come, not from the press, but from members of the public ... [T] he press will ... always feature their complaints not in the least because it is hostile to the profession (for it is not) but purely because such occasions are specially rich in what it calls 'human interest'.[10]

In other words, the source of the 'bad press' of the medical profession was not the media itself, but disgruntled members of the public complaining about substandard medical treatment for which there seemed to be no redress.

Although the establishment of the Public Relations Committee to counter this 'bad press' may seem to have been an inconsequential development, it indicated that the leaders of the AMA had an uneasy suspicion that the issue of health complaints could constitute an Achilles heel for the standing and power of their profession. That suspicion was well-founded; as will become clear in later chapters, it was the issue of patient complaints that eventually led to the destruction of the wall of non-accountability with which successive Medical Practitioners' Acts had surrounded the medical profession in NSW.

However, while the formation of the Public Relations Committee showed that such complaints were having an effect, one result of media critiques was that in the short term, they led to a sympathetic NSW government to surround the medical profession with formidable redoubts to repel consumer complaints.

The closure of health complaints pathways

In line with the Labor government's newfound trust in MM, the Act of 1963 not only placed the handling of complaints entirely in the hands of the medical profession, but also made the registration of such complaints very difficult and their satisfaction practically impossible. The Act specified that any complaints had to be laid before the Medical Registration Board, the unaccountable status of which, dating back 100 years, remained in place. The members of this body were all members of the AMA, but before they considered any complaint, it had to be screened by a three-person, part-time Investigating Committee, one an AMA representative, another a stipendiary magistrate (who headed the Committee) and the third the Director-General of State's Public Health Department (who was generally a medical practitioner and very likely also a member of the AMA) or their nominee.

The Act also stipulated that the hearings of the Investigating Committee were to be held *in camera* (precluding the press from picking up juicy human interest stories), while anyone registering a complaint had to put down a deposit of £5 (the equivalent of at least $50 in 2020) and support their complaint with a statutory declaration. If the Investigating Committee decided that a complaint was 'vexatious or frivolous' or contained false information, the complainant would not only lose their deposit, but could also be fined £100 for making false statements under oath.[11]   If the Investigating Committee did judge the complaint to be genuine and justified, it would be passed on to the Medical Tribunal for final adjudication. There the case would have to be re-argued from scratch by the complainant or their legal representative.

These constrictions of the channels for health complaints ensured that after 1963 the number of complaints which ended successfully for the complainants slowed to a trickle. Whereas the Board of Health had sent about six cases a year to the Medical Tribunal, under the new system, the number of successful cases averaged a little more than one a year over the next decade. Moreover, an analysis of these cases shows that they mostly involved offences relating to the 'infamous conduct' of publicly-visible addiction to alcohol or drugs, not to substandard medical practice.[12]   While the number of registered doctors in NSW rose from 6,658 in 1967[13] in 9,878 in 1972 [14] (i.e. by 32%), there was very little year-on-year variation in the number of actions over the period under review.

That the number of disciplinary cases was extremely low can be appreciated by contrasting it to statistics produced by the Complaints Unit of the Department for Health established in 1984. This was a little over a decade later and it is unlikely that conditions would have altered dramatically over that time period. In 1985-86, its first year of operation, the Complaints Unit received no fewer than 500 written complaints and 200 telephone inquiries.[15]

What is clear is that for two decades after 1963, people who had experienced sub-standard treatment were in the same situation as the Buledelah loggers in the 1930s. The legal pathway for the registration of health complaints was so hedged about with obstacles for complainants that, in practical terms, there was simply no way aggrieved patients could get their complaints redressed or obtain any kind of compensation. The replacement of the words 'infamous conduct' in the Medical Practice Act with the word 'misconduct' in 1973 made no difference to the outcomes of the few disciplinary cases that trickled through the system in the years between then and 1987, when these words and the social constructions behind them were finally eliminated altogether.

What had become increasingly obvious was that those constructions had led to a classic case of regulatory failure. And the reason for that failure had been recognised a long time before in ancient Rome, in fact, when the phrase *quis custodiet hos custodies?* - 'who guards the guardians?' – had been coined. If the purpose of medical regulation had been to safeguard the public interest, the guardians, in the shape of the Medical Registration Board, had been careful to safeguard only the interests of the medical profession. They were able to do this both as a result of the sociological factor of the high status accorded to the profession by the upper classes and sections of the middle class, and also the mundane administrative factor that at the time of the formation of the Medical Board in the earlier 19th century, the rule that bodies exercising delegated governmental powers were responsible to the parliament was unknown. Thus, no doubt due to the high social standing of the medical profession, that Board continued to exercise its almost totally unaccountable power for more than two-thirds of the 20th century.

The choking off of medical disciplinary action during that time created a huge reservoir of frustration and anger against the medical profession which grew exponentially as a result of the Chelmsford Hospital 'Deep Sleep' therapeutic experiments, during which 25 of the 1,430 patients subjected to so-called deep sleep 'therapy' in a hospital in northern Sydney, between 1963 up to the time when it was stopped in 1979, died as a direct result, while large numbers suffered varying degrees of trauma and brain damage.[16] However, the Medical Registration Board took no action against the medical staff of the Hospital until 1985 and, because of the passage of time, no one was ever found guilty of malfeseance. That medical professionals in this case were seen to be literally 'getting away with murder' stoked the fires of public anger and by then, governments had joined in the critiques.

Those rising critiques of the medical profession were part of a cascade of critical literature produced by works such as Ivan Illich's *Medical Nemesis*,[17] Richard Taylor's *Medicine out of Control*,[18] Evan Willis's *Medical Dominance*,[19] and James Le Fanu's *The Rise and Fall of Modern Medicine*. [20] The chorus of critiques of MM undermined its social authority while its status, if not its power, was further challenged by the Holy Grail of state registration being attained as we have seen, by not only other health professional occupations and the UCM modalities of chiropratic and osteopathy but also in Victoria, even by Traditional Chinese medicine.

The consumerist cyclone

While in the early 1960s the Labor Health Minister Sheahan obviously saw health complaints as a nuisance and presided over the 1963 legislation which resulted in them being virtually choked off, 20 years later another Labor Minister for Health, Mr Laurie Brereton, saw health complaints as pure electoral gold. That was one result of the consumerist breezes of the mid-20th century which had led the Medical Association to appoint its Public Relations Committee, becoming a cyclone in the form of what became known as the 'consumer movement'. That had first emerged in institutional form in the United States as far back as 1929 and tardily following that example, the Australian Consumers Association (ACA) was established in 1959. But rather than being the generating force behind the wave of consumerist sentiment which burgeoned over the next ten years, the Consumerist Association, like a surfboarder, merely rode that wave which had obviously been running in powerful although inchoate existence for a long time.

The initial membership of the Consumerist Association garnered from public meetings and other activities, was 500 and these members were the recipients of the first edition of its magazine *Choice* published early in 1960. Writing about that event 25 years later, one of the founder-leaders of the Association, Dr Roland Thorp of the School of Pharmacology at the University of Sydney, stated:

> When those magazines were delivered … subscriptions started to pour in, and our initial print-run of 5,000 was soon exhausted and another 15,000 were ordered. Offers of help came from all sides – we could see that ACA was going to be a huge success.[21]

A decade after the establishment of the Consumerist Association, there were 60,000 subscribers and that number had risen to 100,000 in 1979[22]. This Association ranked as a major organisation of which governments realised they had to take careful note, and that applied in the health sphere as much as in any other.

Here the advent of consumerism was signalled by the formation of the Medical Consumers' Association (MCA) in 1978. Although it never attracted a major membership, one of its leaders, Professor Erica Bates in her book *Health Systems and Public Scrutiny*, claimed that this was 'the most active of consumer groups in Australia and between 1976 and 1978 obtained a great deal of media coverage for its exposure of doctors' high incomes and its complaints at the gradual erosion of the protection afforded to consumers by health insurance'.[23] In 1978 the Medical Consumers Association published a Charter of Patients' Rights and Responsibilities which Bates noted, was praised by the AMA *Gazette* and adopted in a modified form by the Australian Hospital Association.

Governments took a close interest in this mass consumerist movement; after all, there were many more consumers than providers of goods and services, and favouring the former over against latter was in electoral terms, a 'no brainer'. The first visible response of the government in NSW was the passing of the

Consumers' Protection Act of 1969 which established a Consumer Affairs Council composed of consumer representatives who acted in an advisory capacity to government. The Act also set up a Consumer Affairs Bureau (CAB) as a unit within the Department of Labour and Industry, to give advice to consumers and to receive complaints about sub-standard goods and services. In introducing the Act, which established the Department, the Minister, Mr Eric Willis, declared: 'Consumers need help and this is a government responsibility'.[24]

Although the Consumer Affairs Bureau had no regulatory or punitive powers, its activities, like those of the Australian Consumers' Association, evoked an enormous public response. After the first year of its operation, the Bureau reported that 'complaints continue to be received in ever increasing numbers and rate of intake tends to outstrip the growth in staff resources…' The Annual Report of 1972-73 noted that the 6,658 complaints received during the year represented a 63% increase over those of the year before.[25] In 1976, the work of the Bureau was transmuted into that of a fully-fledged department which by 1980 was dealing with 250,000 complaints per annum.[26]

Significantly, Annual Reports of the Department of Consumer Affairs for the years 1978/81 all commented on the increasing number of complaints against doctors accused by their patients of incompetence, unskilled treatment and inadequate services. However, as already pointed out, at the time there was no way in which such complaints could be addressed or redressed.

The spreading net of accountability

While the activities of the Department of Consumer Affairs signalled the beginning of a new approach by government to consumer rights, it was still solely concerned with interactions between consumers and providers in the private sector. But that represented only the first phase of consumerism. The second much less visible, but in many ways profoundly more important phase, was the adoption from the 1970s onwards, of the notion of

Administrative Law, in terms of which government bureaucracies and bureaucrats were also seen to be accountable to the citizenry for actions taken in their official capacities. Administrative Law, in Wilenski's words 'brought judicial power into administration in order to redress the balance of bureaucratic power'. [27]

Through the establishment of government-sponsored and financed agencies such as Ombudsperson's offices, the institution of freedom of information legislation and the establishment of Administrative Appeals Tribunals, it became possible for individual citizens to have their complaints and concerns about governmental actions and decisions taken up and investigated at little or no cost. It thus became possible, for the first time, for members of the public to have their complaints about hospitals and health care institutions investigated. They had also been provided with a state-sponsored champion in their encounters with such institutions.

Just as, if not even more important, was the onset of a third phase of the accountability net which went beyond the governmental sphere to take in the professions. This was evident in a clause of the 1980 Consumer Protection Amendment Act in NSW which enabled the Consumer Commissioner 'to receive complaints about fraudulent or unfair practices by members of the professions, including medical professionals.' This move evoked some heated opposition both outside and also inside the parliament, where Mr K. Rozzoli (Coalition, Hawkesbury) pointed out that the proposal had been opposed unanimously by the professions, and in particular by the Law Society of New South Wales, the AMA, the Australian Hospital Association and the Dental Association, as well as by organizations such as the Council for Civil Liberties. He argued: 'No matter how strongly the Minister may assert that there is no difference between going to the doctor and ... going to the butcher and buying a pound of sausages, there is a considerable difference'.

In response, Health Minister Brereton asked: 'What is so sacrosanct about the so-called professions? Are not consumers entitled to every protection from professionals?' Another participant in the debate, John Hatton (Independent, South Coast) argued:

> In the past ten to fifteen years the professions have come under great scrutiny. Experience has revealed that merely because a person is a professional does not mean that improper practices are beneath him [sic]. This has been made quite clear in the professions of medicine and law. In many instances the improper practices have been evident to an extent that could be described only as shocking. [28]

That these parliamentary critics of professional immunity from investigation did not stand alone was evident from the report of the NSW Law Reform Commission which had averred that 'The … proposition that professionals can be trusted always to put the public interest ahead of sectional professional interests, is one which few people will accept today'.[29] Such statements reflected the fact that the aura of 'priestly mystery' with which the medical profession had defended itself through the use of mumbo-jumbo terminology such as 'infamous conduct' was rapidly disappearing.

The end of MM's political power

Social and political developments such as those described above betokened that not merely a wind but a cyclone of changed thinking was blowing through the Australian community. More evidence of that was provided by the 1972 election of the Labor government in the Commonwealth sphere, bringing to an end 23 years of rule by conservative Liberal/National Party Coalitions.

The reign of Labor administrations under Prime Minister Gough Whitlam over the next three years was tumultuous. Still, towards the end of his tenure Whitlam was persuaded by health advocates such as Dr John Deeble to pass legislation instituting for the first time near-universal governmentally-funded health insurance in the form of the 'Medibank' legislation. That move was fiercely opposed by the AMA and the conservative Parliamentary Opposition who forced Whitlam's administration to a 'double dissolution' election in which all seats in both the Upper and Lower Houses of the Commonwealth Parliament had to be contested. Whitlam won that election but his victory proved to be short-lived; six weeks later he and his government was dismissed by the Governor-General in the famed 'Constitutional Crisis' in 1975. In the ensuing election Whitlam was defeated and over the next few years, conservative Coalition governments, much more sympathetic to and reflective of majority MM opinion, proceeded to dismantle Medibank piecemeal.

Still, the AMA's opposition to Medibank not only caused resentment among the general population, but also sparked an internal revolt among younger, more radically-minded medical professionals who did favour the introduction of Medibank and when they formed the Doctors' Reform Society in 1973, that was a pointer to the decay of the social authority of MM in the political field.

That decay became glaringly evident in NSW, where the heavy defeat of Whitlam's Labor Party in the Commonwealth sphere in 1975 was not duplicated in the NSW State election of 1976. That election brought to power a radically-minded Labor Government headed by Mr Neville Wran. One of its most radical members was Brereton mentioned earlier, who was appointed Minister for Health in 1983. He epitomised the way in which the Labor Party had resumed its ancient hostility to the medical profession and particularly the AMA. The roots of that hostility can very likely be traced to the suspicion and rejection of MM and the medical profession by the majority of the working and middle classes in NSW in the 19th century, outlined in Chapter 2.

Brereton initiated some historic moves, although probably nobody at the time or since realised just how epochal they were, ending as they did, the totally non-accountable status of the Medical Registration Board. One of these changes was to the way its members were appointed. These had customarily been nominated by the AMA and later, also by the Royal Colleges, governments merely rubber-stamping these nominations.

After taking office, Brereton quickly launched moves to break the control of the medical profession by piloting through the parliament an amendment to the Medical Practitioners' Act (No. 177, 1983) which for the first time in its 150 year history, made the Medical Registration Board accountable to the State Parliament. That meant it had lost the completely autonomous status it had enjoyed ever since 1838 and had become just one more of the innumerable statutory authorities in NSW.

Another important change resulting from this Act was the way it not only increased the membership from 9 to 11, but it also specified that two members should be nominated by the Minister on the grounds that they were 'conversant with the interests of patients as consumers of medical services.' Among those he appointed under this heading was Ms Philippa Smith, who at the time was managing director of the newly constituted Health Complaints Unit (the crucial role of which will be detailed in Chapter 8), while he also appointed Dr Marcus Einfeld, an outspoken champion of human rights, as the legal representative.

In 1987 Brereton introduced another set of amendments to the Medical Practitioners' Act which were not only the most extensive since 1963, but also brought about the most radical change to the system of medical regulation since 1901. The Act created an entirely new disciplinary system in terms of which 'infamous conduct' or 'misconduct in professional respect' was replaced by a clause in which professional misconduct was defined as including 'any conduct that demonstrates a lack of adequate (i) knowledge (ii) experience (iii) skill (iv) judgement; or (v) care. In other words, incompetence and negligence on the part of individual physicians or health institutions now constituted punishable offences in terms of the law. The Buledelah hospital and its doctor would not have fared well under this legislation.

MM in transition

The way the Medical Registration Board, the central bastion of MM and also MM practitioners, were stripped of their legal powers in NSW, was just one aspect of the overall decline of the power and influence of MM towards the end of the 20th century. It also began to suffer a loss of its social authority in the eyes of not only of the general population, but those of the younger members of the medical profession. Thus MM was suffering a 'hollowing out' as those who in earlier decades might have been its faithful foot soldiers began to desert its fighting ranks. Among these 'deserters' were a good numbers of physicians who had begun to study and use UCM modalities on a scale which led Pirotta in 2003 to state on the basis of extensive research that 'there is evidence in Australia of widespread acceptance of acupuncture, meditation, hypnosis and chiropractic by GPs.'[30] That statement indicates the onset of what came to be known as 'Integrative Medicine,' in terms of which some medically trained members of the medical profession were incorporating aspects of UCM into their practice of MM.

It was doctors such as these, as well as UCM practitioners, who in 1992, established the Australian Integrative Medicine Association (AIMA) which as its name implies, sought to integrate MM practice with that of UCM. As recorded by Pirotta, numbers of medical doctors and even specialists, were incorporating UCM modalities such as those specified by him, into their practice. Unlike the AMA, the AIMA did not restrict its membership to practitioners of either MM or UCM, but was and is open to anyone interested in integrative medicine.

In the early years of the 21st century, the AIMA gained a notable recruit in the person of Dr Kerryn Phelps, who at the time was president of the AMA (she became the first female incumbent of that post when she was elected to its presidency in 2002). Her move into the AIMA was a result of a life-threatening episode she experienced apparently as a result of her taking hormone replacement therapy, which her treating doctor told her she needed to take with blood-thinning warfarin. But that near-death experience with drug-induced illness 'fueled her inclination to question some mainstream therapies such as HRT which she later saw as an example of how orthodox medicine can go awry at huge cost in death and disease'.[31]

Yet this was not Phelps' first encounter with UCM; that she had been familiar with it over a long period was evident in the way that while she was president of the AMA, she was a driving force in the moves by the AMA which resulted in the publication of its epochal 2002 and 2012 position papers on UCM described below.[32] In 2001, in an article in the *Weekend Australian*, she had argued that 'as evidence emerges that some complementary medicines are effective, then it becomes ethically impossible for the medical profession to ignore them', further pointing out that 'around 17,000 complementary medicinal products are approved for marketing in Australia'.[33] Later she became not only a member of the AIMA described above, but also served as its president between 2009 and 2012.

However, despite gaining recruits such as Phelps, and although it has never been enumerated by the AIMA, its national membership seems to have grown only slowly in the 25-odd years after its founding. Thus it presented little or no challenge to the membership of the AMA which, standing at present at around 8,000 in NSW alone and 30,000 nationally, still makes it the most powerful and highly regarded voice of the health care field both in NSW and in Australia as a whole.

The AMA changes course

But it is that strength that made the 2002 publication of a Position Paper on complementary medicince by the AMA an extraordinary event. If that Paper did not betoken surrender, then it did constitute the running up of a flag of truce in the long 'war' between MM and UCM. Although it covered several pages, the crucial nature of that Paper was summed up in its Point 1, which read:

> The AMA acknowledges the growing use of complementary medicines and therapies by the Australian population [and] recognises that evidence based aspects of Complementary Medicine are part of the repertoire of patient care and may have a role in mainstream medical practice. [34]

Perhaps because of the lack of a long historical perspective, the ephocal nature of this statement was little remarked on. Yet this was the first time since the formation of its predecessor the British Medical Association in 1878 that the AMA, the leading standard bearer of MM, had shown anything but unremitting hostility to UCM. Moreover, one of the most radical aspects of this paragraph is its recognition that UCM, like MM, was including evidence based approaches in its therapies.

However, it was superseded by another AMA Position Paper in 2012 that also recognised that 'evidence-based aspects of complementary medicine can be part of patient care by a medical practitioner'. The paper urged that 'medical practitioners should have access to education about complementary medicine in their undergraduate, vocational and further education to provide advice to patients'.[35] Once again in historical perspective, that statement was an epochal one. The demand in this Paper that UCM practitioners and their activities be subject to 'appropriate regulation' merely indicated that the AMA was not yet aware of the extent of the advances in this medical regulatory sphere which were only slightly less epochal.

The AMA Position Papers of 2002 and 2012 reflected not only a new willingness in MM ranks to recognise the validity of the claims made by UCM proponents, but also constituted an acknowledgement of the decline of MM's social authority as a whole. One of the clearest statements of that phenomenon was articulated by Dr Simon Spedding in the *Medical Journal of Australia* in 2012 when he wrote:

The debates about conventional versus complementary medicine expose how out of touch the medical profession is with the views of government and people about complementary medicine. Now it forms a small proportion of all health professionals registered under the Australian Health Practitioner Regulation Agency (AHPRA), while complementary therapists provide half of health consultations and the public spends almost three times as much on complementary medicine ($3.5 billion) as it spends on prescribed medicines directly ($1.3 billion). Our profession's influence on health policy has been compared with "an ineffective chorus muttering on the edge of the stage about keeping things the way they were."[36]

A mixed metaphor best describes the situation outlined by Spedding: his words constitute a very vivid reflection of the 'state of play' in the 'war' between UCM and MM at that stage. And while the period between the passing of the Medical Practitioners' Acts of 1938 and that of 1987 encompassed the rise and fall of the unchallenged power of MM, Spedding's summation also indicates that these had contributed to the remarkable changes which had occurred in the UCM sphere in the same period and which are recorded in the next chapter.

The end of the Medical Registration Board

Since so much attention has been focused on what had been the central bastion of MM power, the Medical Registration Board in NSW, it seems worthwhile recording the circumstances of its final disappearance. This came about as a result of the Commonwealth government initiating a radical change to the regulation of a range of health modalities, in terms of which responsibility for that function was transferred from the States to a new, centralised body called the Australian Health Practitioners' Regulation Agency (AHPRA), the membership of which is set out in Appendix 1. With agreement of the States, that body was made responsible for the implementation of the 'National Registration and Accreditation

Scheme' which began operating in 2010 and which was designed to iron out the inconsistencies and anomalies resulting from the registration of medical and paramedical practice being enforced by the eight different jurisdictions which comprised the Commonwealth of Australia.

Long before that however, the NSW Medical Registration Board's power over the disciplining of errant medical practitioners had been diluted by the institution of a system of 'co-regulation' in terms of which it shared that function with a new agency, the NSW Health Care Complaints Commission (HCCC), the establishment of which is detailed in Chapter 8. Working in tandem with the Complaints Commission proved difficult for the Medical Registration Board, which according to Andrew Dix, its then Registrar, increasingly felt itself to be sidelined and even bullied by the HCCC.[37] That unhappy experience was finally ended in 2010 when AHPRA began functioning and when, after operating for 170 years, the existence of the Medical Registration Board of NSW was finally terminated. It was replaced by a body called the NSW Medical Council, the membership of which was drawn from the ranks of medical professionals in the State but which had nothing like the power or influence of the NSW Medical Board which dated back to 1838.

CHAPTER 6

UCM - survival and growth, 1938-2008

It can be deduced that UCM was not considered significant during the mid-20th century decades, from the fact that there was still no widely accepted collective noun for it. In 1964 Brian Inglis, a British medical writer, had attempted introduce such a term when he gave the title of *Fringe Medicine* to his substantial book on UCM published in that year. That contained detailed descriptions of all the practices such as chiropractic, osteopathy, naturopathy, herbalism, acupuncture and homeopathy which would shortly come to be known under the collective noun of 'alternative medicine'.[1]

That this term came to be increasingly used from the 1970s onwards, indicated that 'fringe medicine' had failed to gain wide acceptance. Yet while according to the Meriam Webster Dictionary the term 'alternative medicine' began to be used from 1977 onwards,[2] the leading Australian journalist Adele Horin, in 1978 in writing one of the earliest articles on UCM in *The National Times*, used 'fringe medicine' interchangeably with 'alternative medicine'.[3] It was the latter term however, which came to be exclusively used for UCM.

Still, being been deprived of its direct political power and seemingly having no academic or media recognition, did not mean that UCM practice shrank and disappeared in NSW after 1938. If the prohibition of advertising by the Medical Practitioners' Act of that year was meant to suppress the practice of UCM, it failed to do so. Although increasingly less class-based, in fact as argued later, there are strong indications of its continuing and copious use in the years following WWII when the practice and power of MM was at its height and that of UCM seemingly at its nadir.

One of the most telling items of evidence of the widespread practice of UCM came from the NSW Labor Minister of Health Bill Sheehan in 1956. In that year he made what can be termed as a *seminal statement* to the Legislative Assembly (the Upper House) because it laid down the basic policy guidelines which would be followed by NSW governments from that time until the present day:

> Strangely enough, whenever the activities of … so-called 'quacks' have been exposed and demands made that their activities be restricted or banned, the Health Department … received numerous protests that they should not be interfered with. It is felt that a complete prohibition of the activities of numerous unregistered persons who claim to be able to treat diseases would be difficult to enforce and would result probably in the adoption of various subterfuges to defeat it.

Two important points emerge from this statement. Firstly, Sheehan's government was declaring that it had no intention of trying to suppress UCM – to 'put down quackery'. The political costs of doing that were obviously adjudged to be too high and they were to become even higher as the 20th century wore on. The unspoken rider however, was that the government had no intention of trying to exercise any kind of control over the considerable area of medical practice represented by UCM. Although this approach was to change dramatically in the 21st century, governments even then as we shall see, still kept the practice of UCM at arms' length.

Here it can be said that Sheehan's 1956 statement betokened that the NSW government (both the politicians in parliament and the health bureaucracy) saw the practice of UCM as what on early maps was called *terra incognita* – unexplored or unknown territory - about which they had little or no knowledge and even less idea about what they could do to establish or exercise control over practice-standards. Unlike MM, the exclusion of UCM from recognised tertiary institutions for most of the 20th century meant there were no measurable standards by which its practice and practitioners could be judged or disciplined if they harmed or defrauded any of their patients. Moreover, no UCM modality had a controlling body like the MM registration boards with power to act against miscreant practitioners.

Despite these legal shortcomings, what was most notably evidenced by Sheehan's 1956 seminal statement was that UCM continued to enjoy a good deal of recognition and practice in the form of widespread use in the population. This is not surprising. As we have seen UCM was so widely practised in NSW in the 19th and early 20th centuries that its adherents dominated the Lower House anyway, of the NSW parliament. Even though party discipline spelled the end of that control, those UCM-supporting MPs who so passionately argued against the passage of the 1938 Medical Practitioners' Act as well as their supporters, were never likely easily to change their opinions after that Act was passed. This in turn betokened that the historical strength of UCM among the populace of NSW, even if less class-based, was equally unlikely simply to disappear.

While after 1938 the political dimensions of the MM/UCM clash dwindled to practically nothing in NSW, one important development which was to impact this area was the establishment and growth of organisations and associations of UCM practitioners. Those organisations listed below constituted a new feature of the practice of UCM; in the 19th and early 20th centuries such organisations were largely lacking, the followers of UCM at that time constituting simply a powerful but inchoate mass.

In fact it seems that not until 1919 did the first UCM organisation, the Naturopaths and Herbalists Association of Australia, appear on the scene.[4] What is important about the list below, extracted from the Webb Report of 1977 (much simplified from what appears in the Report), is not so much the names of the organisations, but their founding dates because those dates indicate that during the period the eclipse of UCM's visibility in the political, media and academic spheres in the mid-20th century, its practice both in NSW and Australia as a whole, was not only surviving, but was actually strengthening and expanding.

Organisation	Founding date
Australian Institute of Homeopathy	1936
Australian Chiropractors' Association	1938
Australian Osteopathic Association	1941
The National Association of Naturopaths	1946
The Institute of Natural Health	1965
The New South Wales College of Osteopathic and Naturopathic Sciences	1965
The Edward Bach Society of New South Wales	1967
Association of Traditional Health Practitioners	1968
School of Herbal Medicine	1974
South Pacific College of Natural Therapeutics	1974
Association of Natural Health Practitioners	1975 [5]

The formation of these organisations from the mid-20th century onwards might have represented the reaction of UCM proponents to the increasing adoption by MM - as outlined in Chapter 5 - of scientific epistemologies and methodologies which were being applied with considerable success. That would have constituted a major challenge to UCM modalities and the formation of the organisations listed above might indicate a consciousness among their practitioners of a need to systematise and organise their therapeutic practices and the intellectual underpinnings of their various modalities.

The most significant aspect of UCM organisations was not their mere existence: it was rather that they also began to establish training and educational institutions for those who wanted to become practitioners of their particular modality. By 2008, as recorded by Baer, a search of the internet

> ...revealed 26 natural therapies or complementary medicine colleges, four acupuncture/Chinese medicine colleges, two herbal medicine colleges, three homeopathic colleges, 12 massage/bodywork colleges, two reflexology and 6 miscellaneous colleges. [6]

That count he wrote, probably did not exhaust the listing of private complementary medicine colleges in operation at that time.

The quality of the programs provided by these training institutions proved crucial during the 1970s when official recognition of particularly chiropractic, osteopathy and naturopathy began to be considered by both the Commonwealth and State governments. The quality of their training courses and also the validity of their epistemological and intellectual underpinnings came under rigorous governmental/academic scrutiny and not many passed these tests. However, the two modalities which did pass, chiropractic and osteopathy, attained the Holy Grail of full regulatory recognition. But as will be related in Chapter 7, while instituted in NSW in 1978, the initiative had come from the Commonwealth and not the State governments.

UCM's recovery: (1) changing ideas

The later 20th century was a period of intellectual earthquakes, of huge changes in and challenges to thinking about societal issues in Australia as much as anywhere else. These most notably included the anti-Vietnam war movement, the feminist movement, the environmental movement and the emergence of the demands of the Aboriginal population for land rights and political recognition which culminated in their recognition as full citizens of Australia in 1967. UCM was also to ride on this tide of sweeping societal change which strengthened it and moved it towards greater social and political acceptance. But in the second half 20th century, it was no longer economic/class factors but rather sociological developments that became a major if not the major force influencing the course of the 'war' between MM and UCM, and it is to these we now turn.

While it can be deduced from Shelton's seminal statement of 1956 that UCM was being widely used in the mid-20th century, this cannot be supported by reliable statistics based on either official or non-official records. What seems to be true however, is that its usage was not only widespread but began to expand ever more widely particularly from the late 1950s onwards. One reason for that was a general reaction against MM and its practices such as those recorded in the previous chapter. As Lloyd et al recorded in 1993:

> Disenchantment with allopathic medicine and its associated delivery systems has been evident in many industrialised countries since the late 1960s... A better educated and less-accepting public has become disillusioned with experts in general and increasingly sceptical about science and empirically-based knowledge. The high standing of doctors has been eroded in consequence.[7]

Many factors contributed to this development, but perhaps one of the most important was the decline of standing of the medical profession caused among other things by popular resentment of the way the satisfaction of health complaints had been choked off, particularly in NSW. Yet this was only one factor in an evolving situation in which UCM emerged from its post-1938 eclipse.

Another powerful factor was the emergence of the consumer movement and its recognition by governments. Equally significant was a purely sociological factor - the advent of post-modernist philosophy which exercised a powerful influence on the collective consciousness of Western countries anyway, from the 1960s to well into the 21st century. Although the definition and meaning of post-modernism has been widely and vigorously contested, a good working definition was supplied by Siapush when he delineated those influenced by its tenets, as people who

> ... regard nature as benevolent, hold anti-science sentiments, believe in a holistic view of health, reject authority, believe in individual responsibility for achieving good health, and hold consumerist attitudes.[8]

Siapush probably overstated his case when he claimed that those under the influence of post-modernism rejected authority, particularly that claimed by MM. Rather, in the words of Rayner et al, 'post-modernity/late modernity is marked not by a rejection of authority but by a pluralism of authority'.[9] Those acting, even if unconsciously, in terms of 'post-modernity', did not reject scientific medicine as such; rather they saw it as only one of many types of authority and regarded other claimants to authority such as the proponents of UCM as equally 'authoritative' and thus felt that their nostrums could be followed without qualm. This was reflected in the three-city study of Boven et al on 'Current patients of alternative care' undertaken for the Webb Committee in 1977, which reported that the respondents

> ... generally appeared to have a trial and error approach to obtaining care. They commonly visited a variety of traditional practitioners and, when these failed to satisfy them, turned to less traditional forms of help.[10]

In 2012, in writing about the 'postmodern thesis,' in the early 21st century, Coulter and Willis noted that

> ... as social change (also involving globalisation) has accelerated, faith in the ability of science and technology (including medicine) to solve the problems of living had declined. Societal trends towards individualism seem to us to have influenced healthcare trends, with

individuals being less prepared to accept traditional authority such as doctors, and seeking greater levels of control and empowerment over their lives (a trend fuelled by the Internet).[11]

Other studies of the clientele of UCM practitioners recorded the same phenomenon. Not that those who embarked on this kind of post-modern 'therapy shopping' would have consciously seen themselves as 'post-modernists'; in fact, it is likely that a majority had never heard of post-modernism as such.

However influenced by a multiplicity of sources, they absorbed the *zeitgeist* of the times from sources such as those listed in a 2001 study of UCM usage in a NSW rural community, where influences on thinking were listed as friends, family, newspapers and magazines, television/radio, the co-workers of those who were employed and in the case of over 20%, even by orthodox medical practitioners.[12] Moreover, around this time asserted Eastwood, there was 'increasing public disillusionment with scientific medicine,' and that its limitations were becoming apparent to consumers.[13] His research on a small sample of Australian GPs

> ... suggests that there is also a degree of dissatisfaction with traditional biomedicine and its therapeutics, perceived as limited to symptom treatment, limited efficacy in any chronic conditions, overly bureaucratic and institutionalised, too dependent on drugs and not conducive to satisfying and effective healthcare.[14]

Feelings such as these and the resultant strengthening of UCM in terms of its acceptance and growth in the population during the final decades of the 20th century, can be seen in the steady increase in its usage as recorded particularly in scholarly literature. Thus, while in 1983 Wiesner calculated that 8 percent of professional health consultations were with UCM practitioners,[15] a little over a decade later, the Commonwealth Department of Health and Family Services estimated that 57 percent of Australians were using UCM.

In 1993, according to another academic study by McClennan & Taylor, Australians were spending twice as much on alternative medicines 'as patient contributions to all classes of pharmaceutical drugs.'[16]

Another reflection of the advance of UCM were statistics emerging from the 2008 census, which recorded that the number of UCM therapists in 2006 was 80% higher than the number in 1996 and that 'the number of people visiting a complementary health professional (most commonly a chiropractor, naturopath or acupuncturist) increased by 51% in the ten years to 2005'.[17] By 2011, Armstrong et al calculated, 'in a given year, two in every three Australian adults are estimated to use at least one CAM product ... and one in four are estimated to use a CAM service ...[18], while five years later, i.e. in 2016, Reid et al noted that some of the highest utilisation of UCM in any country in the world was in Australia.[19] In 2017 on the basis of their research, Von Conrady and Bonney recorded in The Australian Family Physician that : 'The majority of Australians use complementary and alternative medicine', asserting that that it had 'become an established part of healthcare for many Australians.'[20]

Yet an important gloss on that finding is provided by research into UCM usage which has led several authors to come to same conclusion as Weir et al.

> It appears that the primary consumers of complementary medicine in Australia are relatively affluent individuals who can afford to pay for it either out of pocket or have part of their expenses covered under a private health plan.[21]

The same thought was expressed recently in an editorial in the journal Advances in Integrative Medicine which asserted:

> In Australia it has long been known that users of complementary and integrative (CIM) approaches to healthcare tend to be more affluent, better educated and

otherwise more socio-economically advantaged than other users.[22]

Yet it seems unlikely that such a thin population stratum was responsible, as found by Reid et al, for the highest utilisation of UCM in any country in the world. One possible explanation for the measurements of Weir and other authors such as Willis[23] and Baer is that, like Bruck in the 1880s, they only took into account the clientele of UCM practitioners and did not include 'informal', self-medicating users of UCM, such as those described by Armstrong et al who on the basis of their extensive study published in 2011 stated:

> The use of complementary and alternative medicines (CAM) is now commonplace in Australian society. In a given year, two in every three Australian adults are estimated to use at least one CAM product (e.g. vitamin or mineral supplements or herbal remedies) and one in four are estimated to use a CAM service (e.g. acupuncture, massage, chiropractic therapy). [18]

This is line with Wannan's observation of the early early 20th century, that a large amount of unrecorded usage of UCM continued into the later decades of the century as people, encouraged by the increasing attention paid to UCM by both popular and serious media, continued to use UCM therapies in an unrecorded fashion.

Moreover, in their study of complementary and alternative medicine providers in NSW, Wardle *et al* found that 'complementary and alternative providers form a significant part of the health care system in rural NSW'[24] and that there was also high usage of UCM by rural populations, who are unlikely to be more 'socio-economically' advantaged than other users. The same would be true of the 83% of Australians diagnosed with cancer who use 'some form of complementary medicine and therapy.'[25]

Although seemingly not central to the political issues of the 'war' between UCM and MM, it might be noted that the much longer time perspective of the present work shows that the greatest support of UCM in the 19th and early 20th centuries in NSW, certainly did not emanate from the 'affluent, better-educated and socio-economically advantaged classes'. Just the opposite in fact, as was demonstrated in the voting patterns of the NSW parliament.

The reversal of this situation is attributable not only to the reasons advanced in Chapter 4 for the decline of middle and working-class use of UCM, but also to the provision of subsidised low-cost pharmaceuticals by the Commonwealth government in the form of the Pharmaceutical Benefits Scheme introduced in 1947. The same effect might have been created by the introduction in the last decades of the 20th century of the Commonwealth government's Medicare scheme which provided semi-universal free health coverage. This could have significantly eroded the use of relatively expensive UCM treatments by lower socio-economic groups, although as argued above, it is unlikely to have altogether eliminated their use by such groups.

And yet, the inroads into the numerical superiority by UCM users and supporters would have been counterbalanced by the ability of those in the 'affluent, better-educated and socio-economically advantaged classes' to wield political influence. A prime example of that is Prof Kerryn Phelps whose accession to the ranks of UCM proponents described elsewhere, resulted in the official attitude of the AMA to UCM being radically altered.

Moreover, one by-product of the widening use of UCM was the financial power it put into the hands of companies producing non-pharmaceutical medications. The most notable of these was and is the Blackmores company, an old family business founded by the father of the current owner, Marcus Blackmore. It was important enough to be subject of a major article in the *Business Review Weekly* in 2006, which noted that its share price had improved from $7.80 in 2004 to $14.35 in 2006.[26] Less than 10 years later at a price $200 each, Blackmore shares were one of the four most expensive on the

Australian Stock Exchange. On the basis of this financial strength, Blackmores would be responsible for a significant UCM advance into the academic sphere.

UCM's recovery (2): Media Attention

The year of 1979 has been chosen to mark the start of the re-establishment of UCM's social authority in the media sphere because that was the date when alternative medicine received its first-ever mention in the *Medical Journal of Australia (MJA)*. Written in reaction to a descriptive article on UCM in the *New England Journal of Medicine,* the *Medical Journal of Australia* did not use either 'fringe' or 'alternative medicine' but in its title referred to '(W)holistic Medicine', which became 'holistic medicine' in the text of the editorial itself. Significantly while the MJA had paid no attention to UCM by this date, none the less the editorial noted that 'The holistic movement is flourishing in Australia', yet more evidence that UCM had by no means disappeared in the decades between 1940 and 1980.[27]

Yet as evident from literature searches, that fact was unrecorded in both scholarly and popular media in the 1960s and also much of the 1970s. *The Medical Journal of Australia* article signalled that the long dearth of both the scholarly and popular articles on UCM had ended. This was confirmed In the October 1983 edition of the *Current Affairs Bulletin* entitled simply 'Alternative Medicine,' in which Wiesner recorded that:

> In the past ten years information about the natural therapies has appeared with increasing frequency and in increasing volume in the print media in books, magazines and newspapers. More recently, documentaries and commentaries have appeared on radio and television and have occupied peak evening viewing times.[15]

As related above, the MJA's 1979 article on '(W)holistic medicine' marked the beginning of the recovery of attention to UCM in scholarly media. In fact, the 1980s saw the beginnings of a flood of such articles based academic research and field work. [28] [29] [6, 11, 18, 30, 31] These emphatically established the strong presence of UCM in NSW and Australia as a whole and also betokened its advance into the academic sphere.

UCM's recovery (3). Academic advance

Indicative of an increasingly favourable climate in the academic world was the acceptance by the University of New South Wales in 1983, of the doctoral dissertation of Diane Wiesner entitled *Professionalisation Under Domination. The Natural Therapies in Australia.* Her thesis was that MM had blocked both official and unofficial recognition of UCM and its practitioners in Australia who, she argued, were just as deserving of recognition as the practitioners of MM. But for our purposes, the most valuable contribution of her work was the way in which she tabulated the basic theoretical and practical differences between MM and UCM. It is worthwhile reproducing these in full because they illustrate the 'state of play' at the time and also illuminate much of the discussion in the following chapters.

The objections of MM to UCM Wiesner wrote, were based on the following:

1. The basic assumptions of alternative medicine are not scientific

2. Treatments and remedies used by alternative therapies lack evidence from reliably conducted and reproducible tests under controlled conditions

3. Remedies used by alternative practitioners are not standardised and vary in quality and action from batch to batch.

4. Alternative practitioners have inadequate knowledge and training for the responsibilities they assume – e.g. diagnosis.

5. Alternative practitioners may be able to identify and treat ill

health, but should do so only under medical supervision or with the approval of a practitioner of conventional medicine.

Points 1-4 number among the major accusations made by proponents of MM in the present day, who reject UCM. Over against this according to Wiesner, alternative therapists contended that:

1. In contrast to orthodox medicine, alternative systems are holistic, i.e. they aim to treat the whole person, not just specific symptoms and sites.

2. Alternative therapies and natural remedies are the result of a long history of improvisation and development through clinical practice. Any deficiency in evidence is presently being redressed by a scientific research program to authenticate methods.

3. Alternative remedies are gentle, naturally-based and non-toxic. They show minimal, if any, side effects because they are presented in the naturally-occurring form which the body can easily handle.

4. Alternative practitioners undergo thorough and exhaustive training in theory and clinical practice of their specialities.

5. Alternative practitioners can identify illness and from diagnoses can order and provide treatment; should there be underlying medical problems, they have adequate knowledge to refer the patient to a medical doctor for more extensive tests.[32]

It might be remarked that points 4 and 5 were wishful generalisations: as will be related later, the members of the Commonwealth's 1974 Webb Committee of Inquiry into UCM were not at all impressed with the training particularly of naturopaths which they found to be very weak and disorganised. That they did not give naturopathy the same kind of endorsement that they had given to the UCM modalities of chiropractic and osteopathy meant that to date there has never been any direct official recognition of naturopathic practice in Australia.

Still, Wiesner's use of the word 'holistic' under Point 1 is important because it constituted a UCM riposte to the MM accusation that UCM therapeutic approaches were suspect because, as can be seen from Wiesner's Points 1 and 2 above, they were not derived from peer-reviewed scientific research. On their part, UCM supporters accused MM of being 'Cartesian' in that its practitioners, like the 16th century philosopher Rene Descartes ('I think, therefore I am'), divided mind and body in their therapeutic approaches and tended to see the body in a mechanistic way[33] and being wholly concerned with physical pathologies failed to take the whole 'patient-person' including their social, mental and psychological states, into account.

The word 'holism' had been coined by the South African statesman/philosopher Jan Christiaan Smuts in his book *Holism and Evolution* published in 1925. Although health issues were very far from the main thesis of the book, Wiesner's 1983 use of the word 'holistic' reflects the spread and acceptance of its use particularly by proponents of UCM. They claimed that their therapeutic approaches were and are based on a philosophical position which involves the *whole* person, mind as well as body, over against what they saw as the Cartesian approaches of MM which often failed to take the mental and psychological states of patients into account.

The acceptance of Wiesner's doctoral dissertation by the University of New South Wales in 1983 indicated that UCM was gaining significant authority in the academic field. Conclusive evidence of that in the form of the establishment of academic courses in UCM modalities had to wait for over a decade more, the first such course in NSW being in Traditional Chinese medicine, established in the University of Technology Sydney (UTS) in 1994. Because it was seen to be using a degree of scientific methodology in its teaching, it was initially located in the Faculty of Science but later fell under the aegis of the School of Life Sciences.[34] By 2016 it was a full-blown department with eight staff members as well as two clinicians who ran its clinic and dispensary.

That was followed by the launching of another course in Chinese medicine offered by the new Western Sydney University from 1996 onwards. At that stage this University had no Medical Faculty and says Dr Alan Bensoussan who headed this department, the Vice-Chancellor was very supportive of the formation of what became known as the Centre of Complementary Medicine Research. When the status of Bensoussan's post was elevated to that of full professor in 2003, he was the first academic advocate of UCM to attain that position in NSW.

Their inclusion of UCM in the curricula of these universities also signalled the commencement of the newly introduced concept of evidence-based research into UCM theory and therapies. This was true of the Southern Cross University at Lismore in northern NSW and also at the University of Technology Sydney (UTS), where a powerful research effort embodied in its Australian Research Centre in Complementary and Integrative Medicine (ARCCIM) was founded in 2002.

Perhaps the most extensive evidence-based scientific research of UCM was launched when, on the basis of Prof Bensoussan's Centre, the National Institute of Complementary Medicine (NICM) was established in 2007 with significant funding both from the Commonwealth and State governments. Although the support from governments dried up over the space of a few years, these were replaced by grants from sources such as the Jacka Foundation, the wealth of which was founded on the proceeds of the naturopathic business practice of its founders, Judy and Alf Jacka in Melbourne. That enabled the NICM to expand its staff from about three when it was first launched, to 55 in 2018. Also indicative of the progress of UCM in the academic sphere were the figures produced by Prof Bensoussan who told the Australian Integrative Medicine Association's national conference of 2016 that 'from 2008 to 2013 approximately $31 million was allocated to almost 300 complementary medicine researchers and 160 full time equivalent research students'.

At this point it is not necessary to detail the advance of UCM into the academic sphere other than point out that by 2016, various courses were being offered in 16 Australians universities; eight of these were in NSW and included three professorial chairs. Most notable was the proposed establishment of a chair of Integrative Medicine at the University of Sydney in 2015 with the help of a $1.3m grant from the Blackmores company, although at the time of writing, this post had not yet been filled because the funding offered by Blackmores was not seen to be sufficient. But perhaps this was a stalling tactic on the part of the university betokening that there was still resistance to, if not rejection of UCM. In fact the Blackmores grant could have been expanded tenfold was evident in the grant of $10,000,000 made to the research programs of the National Institute of Complementary Medicine in 2017.

Whatever the reason for stalling the establishment of the chair of integrative medicine, an article published in the *Honi Soit*, the student newspaper of the University of Sydney, stated:

> Even if academics disagree with the practice of complementary and alternative medicine its presence has become overwhelming in the Australia consumer market. According to the National Institute of Complementary Medicine, Australians spend more than $3.billion on complementary and alternative medicine every year. With this expected to grow to $4.6 billion in 2017, mainstream practitioners can no longer neglect teaching students how these medicines work.[35]

Although that line of thinking produced no immediate reaction from the University authorities, none the less it indicated that there had been a huge amount of change in the position of UCM in the 60-odd years following Sheehan's seminal statement of 1956.

And while the attempt to establish the professorial chair in integrative medicine in the University of Sydney had stalled, an evidence-based graduate certificate in complementary medicines began to be offered by the University's Faculty of Pharmacy in 2018. The course co-ordinator Dr Joanna Harnett, asserted that 'the prevalent use of complementary medicines by the Australian population has remained consistently high over the last two decades,' which meant that 'there is an increased need by the professional bodies for pharmacists to provide information that guides the appropriate safe use of these medicines.'[36]

The elusive regulatory Grail

As we have seen in this chapter, from the late 20th century onwards UCM had immensely strengthened its presence in the three crucial spheres of population usage, media attention and tertiary education. These developments represented not only a medical but also a political reality which governments had perlforce increasingly to recognise.

But if the resurrection or UCM practice meant it had ceased to be *terra incognita*, by the early 21st century, governments' lack of power to control the standards of practice in the obviously hugely expanded field of UCM had remained unchanged. The need to ensure public safety by means of regulation in that field became increasingly urgent during the later 20th century as the expansion of UCM usage made it increasingly clear that this 'sleeping dog' was not asleep at all. However, there was no firm indication of whether it was capable of or was in fact inflicting grievous bodily harm both on members of the public and also on the electoral fortunes of whatever party happened to be in government and therefore responsible for public safety, at the time.

CHAPTER 7

Governments change course

Governmental attitudes to UCM swung remarkably between the mid- and late 20th century. At the one extreme, for close on four decades after the passing of the 1938 Act in NSW, its successive governments paid UCM no attention whatsoever even though, as evident from Sheehan's seminal 1956 statement, they were uneasily aware of the existence of this 'sleeping dog'. The decline and apparent disappearance of UCM's standing in the governmental sphere is evident from its complete absence from either official documents or legislation.

That there was little or no consciousness of UCM in this sphere as late as the 1970s was evident in the Parliamentary debates on the first post-1938 legislation that directly affected its practice in NSW. This took the form of a Bill (No 232:1972) which oddly juxtaposed the regulation of cosmetics with that of therapeutic goods, the latter including UCM medications, being sold in the State. The general level of debate on this Bill can be judged from the question of one member, who asked the Minister for Labour and Industry piloting the legislation to

> ...explain the dividing line between cosmetics and therapeutics. When does a cosmetic cease to be a cosmetic and become a therapeutic? I am informed by my wife and other women that I know that cosmetics are generally regarded by all women as therapy.[1]

That brand of crass sexism set the tone for further speeches in the debate, in which speakers devoted practically all their attention to the regulation of cosmetics while largely ignoring therapeutic goods. UCM received no attention at all.

None the less, the expansion of the authority of UCM in the three spheres outlined in the previous chapter as well as the decline in the standing of Mainstream Medicine (MM), did not go unnoticed in either the Commonwealth or the State governmental spheres. Thus, although hostility towards UCM by powerful elements within MM did not decrease, the resurgence of UCM prompted a notable change in governmental attitudes towards UCM in the late 20th and early 21st centuries.

Scholars who have discussed this phenomenon, include both Willis[2] and Coburn. In the latter's view:

> ...biomedical dominance in Australia has been eroding as the federal government and state governments as well as corporations have to come to play a more predominant role in the creation of health policy, which in turn have begun to adopt a greater tolerance for complementary medical systems. This growing tolerance, however, is probably more related to the perception that they are cheaper forms of health care than to the fact they offer competing philosophies of health.[3]

It can be argued however, that the 'growing tolerance' of governments for UCM, was not only due to the possibility of its practice easing the strains on the public purse but also to an extension of the 'Sheehan effect': if it was politically impossible to suppress UCM, it was equally impossible to contain its acceptance by a growing sector of the voting populace in the State.

It must have quickly dawned in party political circles that recognition of that trend could reap rich electoral rewards – and have the opposite effect if they failed to recognise it. If that was the case, it would indicate that electoral factors were as powerful a force in prompting greater governmental acceptance of UCM as the economic factors portrayed by Coburn.

Breakthrough for chiropractic and osteopathy

Changed governmental attitudes to UCM were first evident in the Commonwealth sphere after the election of the radical Whitlam Labor government in 1972. Those changed attitudes were most clearly seen in the case of chiropractic, the origins and epistemology of which are described in Chapter 1. As indicated earlier, its practitioners had established a national association as early as 1938.

An account which appeared in their official journal, *ACO*,[sic] indicates the success of this kind of association in gaining governmental recognition was a result of both its level of organisation and the standards of training it provided for its practitioners. Together, these enabled chiropractic and also osteopathy (also described in Chapter 1) to gain the much sought-after official registration of their practices in both the Commonwealth and State spheres. The way this happened was detailed in an account authored by Edwin Devereux of Sydney, who became president of the Australian Association of Osteopaths and Chiropractors in 1961. Before then he had been a trade union organiser and as a member of the NSW Trades and Labour Council, had been in close contact with the leaders of the Australian Labor Party (ALP) both in NSW and in the Commonwealth spheres of governments.

The election of Whitlam's Labor government in 1972 provided Devereux with opportunities to lobby leading figures who, after being elevated to the Federal cabinet, had the power to change the medical and social landscape. Among these were Bill Morrison, Minister for Science and Dr D.N. Everingham, Minister for Health and also Bill Hayden, Minister for Social Security, later to become leader of the ALP. According to Devereux, after being lobbied, Hayden agreed to introduce a motion at the national conference of the ALP in 1973, calling for official recognition and registration of chiropractors. Devereux reported Hayden as saying: 'You are handling peoples' bodies, so you should be registered.' It was the passing of this resolution according to Devereux which after a complicated process, led in 1974 to the establishment by the Whitlam government of the 'Committee of Inquiry into Chiropractic, Osteopathy and Naturopathy,' under the chairmanship of Professor E.C. Webb, formerly vice-chancellor of Macquarie University in Sydney.[4]

This 'Webb Inquiry' provided the means for chiropractic and osteopathy to attain the Holy Grail of governmental regulation. (Although chiropractic had already gained official registration status in Western Australia in 1964[5] none of the other States had followed that lead.) It was only as a result of exhaustive research into general UCM training and practice that the Webb Committee recommended that chiropractic and osteopathy in particular be granted official registration by all the Australian States.[6] Conversely, as mentioned earlier, the Committee's unfavourable view on the standard and quality of naturopathic training courses (one of which they saw as 'decidedly dangerous[7]), sank any hopes its practitioners may have had of also gaining government-recognised registration courses between that time and the close of this account.

Although Whitlam's Labor government fell in 1975, none the less in the State sphere continuing Labor governments in both Victoria and NSW passed Chiropractic Registration Acts and established Chiropractic Registration Boards in 1978. But while chiropractors and osteopaths were not permitted to assume the title of 'doctor' and could issue only five specialist referrals in a month, they none the less had become the first UCM practitioners to be given this form of official standing by the governments of NSW and Victoria. In other words, these UCM modalities at least, had attained the Holy Grail of S[s]tate registration and regulation in these States, even if the limitations on that regulation meant that this was only a 9-carat Grail.

In Victoria the granting of official registration to Traditional Chinese Medicine (TCM) in 2002, recognised that this form of UCM, long practiced in that and other Australian States, had as a result of Chinese immigration throughout the 20th century, become increasingly prominent and widely used and not only in the immigrant Chinese population. Although Victoria's lead of granting official regulatory registration to TCM was never followed in NSW or anywhere else in Australia, as we have seen TCM 'led the charge' into the academic sphere in NSW and was one of the 12 modalities brought under the aegis of the Australian Health Practitioners Regulatory Agency (AHPRA) described elsewhere which, for reasons related in Chapter 9, elevated TCM to the same regulatory status throughout Australia as chiropractic and osteopathy.

However, long before this, the fact that the growing popularity of UCM had forced changes in government attitudes in the Commonwealth sphere is evident from its creation of the Therapeutic Goods Administration which began operating in 1991 as a regulatory body tasked with ensuring the safety (although not the efficacy) of all pharmaceuticals and other medications sold in Australia. That UCM products were included in the purview of this new body indicated a recognition that they were being used by a growing segment of the population and therefore could not be ignored.

Growing governmental recognition of UCM practice in Australia was also reflected in the calling by the Commonwealth Health Minister of an 'Alternative Medicine' summit in 1996. That was because, in the words of the Parliamentary Secretary for Health, Senator Bob Woods, 'the government could no longer ignore the increased consumer demand for alternative medicine... [8] In this conference, governmental representatives and UCM leaders met face-to-face for the first time, while in 2003 a much sharper focus on UCM was created by the establishment of the Office of Complementary Medicines as a unit within the Therapeutic Goods Administration 'to focus exclusively on the regulation of complementary medicines'.

As can be seen, the words 'alternative' and 'complementary medicine' were being used interchangeably around the last decade of the 20th century and the first of the 21st. That issue was the subject of an article by Coulter and Willis in the *Medical Journal of Australia* in 2004. Entitled 'The rise and rise of complementary and alternative medicine: a sociological perspective' the authors summarised the issue as follows:

> The issue of what to call the C[omplementary] A[lternative] M[edicine] group has important social and political ramifications. To term the group of modalities *alternative* may seem to claim too much for their role in healthcare, but to term them *complementary* may make their role seem secondary to primary health care.[9]

It is to avoid this terminological minefield that, as outlined in the Introduction of this work, the acronym of UCM has been used throughout this work to denote what, in the late 20th and early 21st century, came to be referred to as CAM. As will be appreciated, that term is scarcely two decades old and certainly using it to describe UCM during the 150-odd years prior to 2000 would be historically anachronistic.

Still, what can be seen from the name of the Office of Complementary Medicine, is that by the time of its founding, the acronym CAM had become entrenched in official circles. The creation of this Office had come about as a result of the 'Pan Crisis' of early 2003 which had erupted after the recall of some of the products of Pan Pharmaceuticals, the biggest manufacturer of UCM medications in Australia at that time.

In response, the Commonwealth government moved swiftly to appoint an 'Expert Committee' to investigate whether any Pan products posed a danger to the community. Membership of this committee included public servants active in the health field, representatives of the therapeutic medicine industry and academics. Significantly, among the latter were leading UCM advocates Profs

Alan Bensoussan of the Centre for Complementary Medicine Research at the University of Western Sydney and Prof Steven Myers of Southern Cross University. Their presence reflected that the open hostility or at best, indifference to UCM which prevailed a decade or two earlier, had fallen away and that the Commonwealth government was now giving it explicit recognition. That was evident in the Expert Committee's statement that UCM medicines 'are an important part of the Australian health care system and are used by a substantial proportion of the population both here and overseas'.[10]

The Expert Committee had been tasked with examining and providing advice on 'regulatory controls on the standards, safety and efficacy of complementary medicine ... the education and training of healthcare practitioners' and 'activities to promote an innovative, responsible and viable complementary medicines industry'.[11] The Committee's conclusion that it 'lacked confidence in any of the products manufactured by Pan company', caused the Therapeutic Goods Administration to withdraw Pan's manufacturing licence which in turn led to the company's collapse. But this was just one aspect of the Expert Committee's exhaustive 164-page report, which included a 10-page glossary describing different types of UCM therapies. When it was published in September 2003, it constituted the most complete mapping of the UCM field – terra incognita in Sheehan's day in 1956 - in Australia to that date.

Regulation – a new/old problem

This was not the only map however. In the previous year the NSW government had produced its own account of UnConventional medical practice in the form of a report entitled Regulation of Complementary Health Practitioners. The extensive survey of UCM practice in Australia in general and NSW in particular outlined in this paper, claimed that far from UCM being a 'sleeping dog', it posed serious potential risks for its users, including failure to 'detect serious underlying disease, mental trauma, unsubstantiated claims of therapeutic benefit, sexual misconduct and financial exploitation'.

Yet, as noted by this paper, there was a lack of any effective complaints handling mechanisms for UCM practice and that on that score, apart from admonishing miscreant practitioners, even the NSW Health Care Complaints Commission lacked any power to take action against them. Moreover, according to the NSW paper, there was one major reason for that state of affairs – the lack of any regulation applying to UCM.[12]

That same issue, it may be recalled, had arisen in NSW 150 years before in relation to 'the conduct and safety' of MM practice. The answer became increasingly clear as the 19th century progressed: the regulation of MM by the means described in Chapter 1. In the 21st century the application of that regulatory solution to UCM was blocked by two seemingly insurmountable obstacles, one a formal, legal one and the second a much more political one.

The first legal obstacle was that unlike MM, there were no professional registration boards controlling UCM practice. In MM, the legally established Medical Registration Board had ever since 1901, been empowered to take action against miscreant professionals, leading to them being struck off the Medical Register in extreme cases. The same was true of other Boards established in the course of the 20th century, including, those for Dentistry, Nursing, Optometry and Physiotherapy among others. In contrast in UCM, apart from chiropractic and osteopathy, there were no similar legally established Boards, and while there were a multitude of UCM organisations, these were powerless to take action against miscreant practitioners because their membership was voluntary and they thus had no means of enforcing any kind of discipline against such miscreants.[13]

The second obstacle blocking the introduction of regulation of UCM modalities, which may be described as political, was set out by the 'Expert Committee' when it stated: 'Medical stakeholders opposed to statutory registration for any complementary medicine profession have argued that statutory registration will confer undue recognition on professions whose practices are unproved and that the evidence of harm caused by these professions is insufficient to justify legislation.' In simpler terms, MM was blocking the path to registration by UCM modalities, an interesting historical contrast to the 19th century situation, when UCM supporters in the NSW parliament continuously blocked the registration of MM practitioners. Now according to the Expert Committee 'the boot was on the other foot'. Another formidable obstacle to extending registration to UCM modalities noted by the Expert Committee was that 'with no enforceable barriers to entry to practice, and multiple, separate professional associations representing practitioners' interests, consensus on standards of training is virtually impossible to achieve'.[14]

But while the work of the Expert Committee failed to provide much comfort on the score of registration to UCM, it did make an encouraging observation on another crucial issue, that of research, declaring that 'a viable and innovative complementary medicines industry is dependent on research to underpin the quality, safety and efficacy of the complementary medicines and to develop new products'.[15] Citing the success of the government-funded National Centre for Complementary and Alternative Medicine established in 1992 in the United States, the Committee recommended that a similar UCM research body be established with governmental seed-funding in Australia. Exactly that kind of research body, the earlier mentioned National Institute of Complementary Medicine came into being in 2007 in the University of Western Sydney, based on the platform provided by the Centre for Complementary Medicine Research headed by Professor Alan Bensoussan. It was initially financed by a $6m grant from the Commonwealth Government supplemented by a grant from the NSW government.[16]

The third map

A third great mapping of UCM practice in Australia was produced in 2006 by Profs Bensoussan and Myers together with Dr Phillip Cheras of Queensland University and Dr Margaret Cook, Executive Officer of the Nursing and Midwifery Council of NSW. Demonstrating how high UCM stood in some circles of the NSW government, their report was drawn up under the aegis of the NSW government's Ministry of Science. Entitled *Complementary Medicine Research – a Snapshot,* this report constituted an even more extensive and thorough mapping of UCM practice than that of the 'Expert Committee'. Although many of the statistics and information provided in this report are outdated, none the less much of its delineation of the operations and 'reach' of UCM remain valid and are therefore worth noting because its conclusions have a bearing on the main theme of this work – the control and regulation of UCM.

In the '...*Snapshot'* the authors presented the information and arguments under nine different headings, which are briefly summarised here:

1. *The size and value of the industry:* The estimated value of the UCM industry was reported to be $1.5 billion to $2.5 billion per annum and also to be growing at a rate of 10% per annum.

2. Under 2, *incidence of use* it was reported that an estimated 70% of Australians consumed a UCM product each year and that by 2000 they were spending $1.7 billion per annum on such products, nearly four times what was spent on pharmaceuticals.

3. *Funding sources and profile.* Here it was recorded that 252 UCM research projects funded by seven different agencies into UCM had been undertaken in the years 2000-2004 at a cost of $26.25 million.

4. This section dealt with *research capacity and activity,* recording that 27 centres and 141 individuals had carried out UCM research projects over the previous year, the greatest number (86) being based in NSW.

5. Under the heading of *Workforce Profile,* the report asserted that a good number of practitioners in the MM sphere 'such as nurses and medical practitioners ... use [U]CM in conjunction with orthodox therapy', stating further that that there were 5-8,000

active UCM clinicians 'who provide a small but significant service within the healthcare system and that the number of CM practitioners is continuing to increase'. It was also noted that there were over 100 professional associations representing UCM practitioners.

6. *Regulation:* Here the report noted that with the exception of chiropractic, osteopathy and Traditional Chinese Medicine in Victoria, UCM practitioners were largely self-regulated. However, the same was not true of UCM therapeutic products. 'Australian [U]CM regulations are considered to be the most well-developed in the world,' of particular note being the regulatory activities of the Therapeutic Goods Administration.

7. The report noted under the *integration of complementary and mainstream medicine* 'there is growing acceptance of [U[CM by medical practitioners in Australia and overseas.' In Australia the AMA and the Australian Medical Council acknowledged the increasing use of UCM and recommended a basic understanding of its therapies by the medical profession. Moreover, the Australian College of Nurses 'supports the use of [U]CM by nurses within the limits of their skill and knowledge and supports the attempts of the profession to integrated [U] CM'.

8. On the apparent failure of UCM to operate on the basis of *evidence-based medicine,* the report noted 'it is important to recognise that traditional knowledge in [U]CM disciplines is not simply anecdotal, but a form of empirical knowledge, as is the collective accumulation of individual observations by generations of practitioners, in some cases over hundreds of years'.

9. Under the last heading of *evidence of efficacy, safety and cost-effectiveness* the authors averred that 'scientific literature exists demonstrating that some complementary medicine interventions have a high level of evidence for their effectiveness,' although it was admitted that 'there remains a substantial gap between the current level of usage and the

scientific evidence which supports it.'

On the basis of the evidence set out in the report and also because the Commonwealth did not renew its original grant to the National Institute of Complementary Medicine, its authors argued that there was an urgent need for greater funding of research into the efficacy, safety and cost-effectiveness of UCM. What is significant to the theme of this work is that in making that plea, they also indicated that despite the recognition of UCM in government circles, the ideological war between UCM and MM was raging unabated. The authors added significantly to what Wiesner had advanced 20 years before as to the causes of that war when they stated:

> There is a concern that the lack of government research funding and the focus on funding from industry is leading to an emphasis on pharmaceutical research based on the western bio-medical paradigm ... It was noted that this approach is not consistent with the philosophical base of many C[omplementary] M[edicine] disciplines that do not treat disease as we know it and believe in a whole person approach to healthcare. The lack of funding for whole practice based research considered to be a problem of the current funding focus.[17]

In addition, the feeling among UCM researchers was that

> '...there is a strong bias against complementary medicine research within the peer funding bodies [because] they are exclusively reviewed by those not involved with Complementary Medicine and those who do not share the [its] paradigm.'[18]

Despite its scholarly depth, the ...*Snapshot* produced little further research funding for UCM from the NSW government. In 2006 its Ministry of Science, which had commissioned the report, was abolished. Some comfort came from the Commonwealth sphere in which the Rudd Labor government had come to power in 2007. In announcing to the third international congress on Complementary Medicine Research in Sydney in 2008 that the National Health and Medical Research Council (NHMRC) was to make grants of over $7m for UCM research, the Parliamentary Secretary to the Minister for Health and Ageing, Senator Jan McClucas, declared that UCM research 'represented a substantial repositioning of activity in the Australian health care sector'. Moreover there was 'growing testimony that complementary medicine can make a significant cost-effective contribution to public health in chronic disease-management and in preventative care'. [19]

While proponents of UCM would have welcomed this kind of explicit governmental recognition, the funding was only the proverbial 'drop in the bucket' compared to the total funding disbursed by the NHMRC. Figures released in 2017 showed that while this body had directed $3.6 billion to MM research projects between 2000 and 2016, only $86 million (2.9%) had gone to grants to similar UCM projects.[20]

Reflecting that in fact UCM got little shrift from the NHMRC, its then Chief Executive Officer Professor Warwick Anderson observed in a speech to the National Press Club in 2015 that 'quackery has come roaring into the 21st century'.[21] Not that the NHMRC is implacably hostile to UCM; rather it evidenced what by then had become a typically governmental attitude of 'acknowledge but don't encourage' attitude as embodied in a clinicians' resource paper it published in 2014 entitled 'Talking with your patients about Complementary Medicine,' on the grounds that 'many Australians report that they used complementary medicine but do not disclose this to their clinicians' and that therefore 'talking about complementary medicine is important'.[22]

Talk however, is not equivalent to money, and UCM has remained in its condition of research funding starvation. In the light of the billions of NHMRC research grants to MM projects cited above, it can be seen that even $10m Blackmores grant to Prof Benssousan's

National Institute of Complementary research of 2017 would not do much more than slightly enlarge the size of its drop in its total research-funding bucket.

The elusive Grail

Yet however meagre governmental financial outlays on UCM research efforts were, they did betoken one important change in governmental attitudes to UCM during the late 20th and early 21st centuries. The 2002 NSW report on the *Regulation of Complementary Health Practitioners,* the 'Expert Committee' report of 2003, and also the extensive 2005 "... Snapshot" report commissioned by the NSW Ministry of Science, meant that for governments, the field of UCM was no longer *terra incognita* - unknown territory.

However, as indicated in especially the 2002 NSW report but also in the other major reports, there was an apparent absence of any kind of regulation designed to safeguard public safety in the field of UCM. That meant that, as was the case with MM in the 19th century in NSW, the practice of UCM in the late 20th and early 21st century was seemingly a chaotic and therefore potentially dangerous free-for-all in which anyone, whatever their training or lack of it, could claim to be a medical practitioner.

Equally evident from the reports was that governments had little or no idea of where they could or should start to remedy this situation. This was despite the fact that for them, finding a way to introduce regulation into UCM practice was as urgent as it was for its practitioners. No one suspected that the pathway to that elusive Grail would be provided by the unlikely phenomenon of patient complaints.

CHAPTER 8

UCM's strange pathway into the medical regulatory system of NSW

Historical happenings very often are not the result of a logical or an ordered progression of events. Instead they are often shaped by unplanned and unanticipated developments which 'come out of left field'. Nothing illustrates that better than the way UCM was brought within the purview of governmental regulation in New South Wales and eventually of much of Australia as a whole.

It might have seemed that the contests over the Holy Grail of regulation in the State sphere ended in 2010. In July of that year, as related in Chapter 6, responsibility for this function which had been exercised by the State and Territory governments for well over a century, was taken over by the new Commonwealth body, the Australian Health Practitioners Registration Authority – AHPRA. As noted earlier, this development finally ended the existence the NSW Medical Registration Board.

That this narrative does not end in 2010 is because the scope of the AHRPA did not extend further than the boundaries of MM and the 13 other professions regulated under the National Registration and Accreditation Scheme (their full list appears in Appendix 1). Yet this legislation did provide a regulatory breakthrough for several . UCM modalities, because it included Traditional Chinese Medicine (TCM) which as noted earlier, had been officially regulated in Victoria since 2002. Since under the new national system of registration it was not possible to contemplate de-regulating such a well-entrenched modality, the best solution was to extend the scope of Victoria's regulatory regime of TCM to the whole of Australia.

That breakthrough for UCM was as important as that achieved by chiropractic and osteopathy thirty years before. And since the scope of TCM also extended to acupuncturists and herbalists acting within its ambit, these modalities insofar as they were considered part of TCM, also fell under the scope of official government regulation. They thus joined chiropractic and osteopathy as officially recognised UCM professions regulated by the AHPRA.

While this development constituted a significant advance in the official recognition of UCM, as will be demonstrated shortly, the great bulk of UCM modalities remained largely unregulated. That meant that the States, and particularly NSW, had been left to grapple by themselves with how to extend Weber's notion of societal 'order and protection' into the sphere of those modalities. Not that that sphere was totally unregulated. As was noted in the final report on the *Options for Regulation of Unregistered Health Practitioners* published by the Australian Health Ministers' Advisory Council in 2013, there were

> ... a range of laws that apply to their practice. ... many practitioners are subject to 'voluntary self-regulation', that is, they voluntarily choose to join a professional association thereby subjecting themselves to the rules of the association. As a condition of their membership, they may agree to abide by a code of ethics, undertake continuing professional development and meet other practice standards. They may have their membership withdrawn by the association for breaches of professional standards. A variety of government and non-government associations that fund or provide health services (such as Medicare Australia, workers' compensation, transport accident insurance, and private health insurance funds) rely on such professional

associations to regulate their members. These 'health payers' may require practitioners to be members of an association in order to become a 'recognised provider' of health services that they fund. Depending on how they are configured, these arrangements for credentialing of practitioners may constitute a type of 'co-regulation'.[1]

Yet five years previous to this report a far more direct and effective solution to the issue of regulating UCM practitioners had been enacted in law in NSW. As will be related in this chapter, the pathway to that regulatory Grail lay through the obscure territory of health complaints – those seemingly insignificant straws-in-the-wind which as noted in Chapter 5, had begun blowing through the NSW health system even before 1938. Understanding the way that happened demands first and foremost an understanding of the way that formal structures for responding to and dealing with health complaints was established in NSW – and eventually most of Australia.

NSW's pioneering health complaints pathway

In the early 1980s, even though the medical profession in NSW had suffered a major fall in public esteem, the official channels for health complaints were still choked and the need to remedy that situation was much discussed in health consumerist circles. One pointer to that was when, in an interview with the NSW Minister of Health Laurie Brereton sometime in the early 1980s, a delegation from the Pensioners and Superannuants Federation raised their difficulties in obtaining redress from doctors with whom they were dissatisfied. They told him that what was needed was 'something like a health Ombudsman'.[3] That indicated that the discourse of administrative law had had been taken up by consumers and when that happened, as noted above, those in government, in pursuit of their own electoral interests, were invariably inclined not only to listen, but also to act.

When Brereton did act, he was seemingly not primarily concerned about health complaints; his stated priority was what he saw as the more pressing issue of medical financial fraud perpetrated by doctors who were over-claiming for their services delivered in terms of the government's universal health insurance system, Medicare. Yet when on April 26, 1983, he announced the establishment of a new body, the chief aim of which was to investigate ' ... the growing number of complaints about fraud and overservicing...' – colloquially known as 'medifraud' - this was not his only concern. In his media release of April 26 1983, he also identified 'the standard of care provided in institutions governed by state legislation' as another major justification for the formation of the new body, although the inclusion of this aim was probably meant to reference to the Chelmsford 'Deep Sleep' disaster rather than being generally applicable to all state healthcare institutions.

Still, indicating the impulsive and ad hoc way in which he had brought the new body into existence, Brereton was still casting around for a director seven months after he made the announcement about its formation.[4] The solution to his search appeared from a direction which, as the last sentence of his April 26 announcement demonstrated, was only peripherally present in his consciousness: health consumer issues. Yet his new body was destined to produce a vehicle for the thinking of the consumer movement which powerfully penetrated the hitherto untouched field of governmental health provision and administration.

This consumerist 'vehicle' appeared in the person of Ms Philippa Smith, who at the time was acting as a consultant to the Health Department. Before this she had gained a reputation as a leading consumer advocate and had played a prominent role in consumer-oriented organisations including the Australian Council for Social Service (ACOSS). When she heard about Brereton's proposal, she obviously saw an opening for the realisation of health consumer interests and thus sent him a memorandum in which she urged that the new body be based on 'a much broader perspective of consumer issues as opposed to the criminal view' and that it 'look at broader issues of quality of care, matters of administration and matters of policy, as they affected consumers'.[5]

Brereton invited her to see him and convinced she was the right person to head the new body, asked her to do so. She readily agreed. But Smith was a typical 'equal health advocate' and for her the question of 'medifraud' was an issue between government and the medical profession. Much more important in her eyes was the question of redressing individual consumer health complaints. Thus once she had been installed as director of the new body, she set about downgrading the 'medifraud' agenda.

Her task in this respect was made easier by Brereton ceasing to be Minister of Health in February 1984, one month after the new body commenced operations. His successor was never as concerned about 'medifraud' as Brereton and Smith's success in imposing different priorities on the new body is evident from a document of 14 May, 1984. There it was reported that during discussions between her, the new Minister and the Secretary and senior officers of the Health Department, it was agreed that the new body would become much more focused on health consumer concerns.[2] Reflecting that emphasis, it was named the 'Complaints Unit' of the NSW Health Department, and when it began functioning early in 1985 it was, as noted earlier, the first unit of its kind anywhere in the world. That reflected the fact that consumer complaints termed above as 'insignificant straws in the wind', now rode on a gale which was radically to affect the struggle between MM and UCM.

The Complaints Unit (from this point forward CU) at last constituted an organisation to which patients who believed they had suffered negligence or been mistreated or injured in government health care institutions, particularly hospitals, could direct complaints. If after investigation by the CU a complaint was found to be valid, it was taken to an appropriate health registration board which in turn could refer the matter to a Medical Tribunal which if it found an accused practitioner guilty of miscreancy, could order their name to be struck off the Medical Register. No doubt the Buledelah loggers would have cheered this innovation, even though its advent came half-a-century too late for them.

From the point-of-view of the present study, it could be said that the establishment of the Complaints Unit closed the regulatory circle for medical practice in NSW. If the basic aim of regulation is to ensure public safety and the Medical Registration Board had been responsible for pursuing that aim, its lack of investigatory powers meant it had never been well equipped to deal with cases of medical failure and malpractice. This gap began to be filled by the CU after 1985.

The NSW innovation represented an idea whose time had come. Before the end of that decade all Australian States and Territories and also New Zealand which of course had also been swept by the post-modernist and consumerist waves of change, had established similar bodies as did the British National Health System. In NSW itself, the CU grew rapidly: by 1987, a mere two years after its commencement, its initial four members of staff had grown to 33 and the annual number of complaints registered with it had increased from the initial 500 mentioned earlier, to 1,946.[6] And whereas in the 13 years between 1966 and 1979, only eight cases had gone before the Medical Tribunal, in 1988 alone the CU took 15 matters to that Tribunal. Also indicative of the expansion of CU activities was that while in 1988 it budget had been just over $1m, by 1993, the number of staff members had risen to 44 and the budget to $2,6m.[7]

The latter figure has an added significance it that it reflected an important politico/ideological development which occurred in the last decades of the 20th century. That development had taken place in the conservative Liberal Party which, together with the National Party under the name of the Coalition, could always be relied on to support the political positions of MM. Thus there were fears among the staff and supporters of the CU after its establishment in 1984, that if and when the Labor Party lost government in NSW, this could also spell the end of the CU.

The fears proved to be groundless; the ideological centre of the Liberal/National Coalition had shifted and the administration of its young new Premier, Nick Greiner elected in 1988, was driven by a 'market   liberal reform strategy'.[8] His government was characterised by a strongly reformist bent and he and the 'dries' in his party who epitomised that thinking, strongly supported demands which had arisen from the consumer and administrative law movements for political and professional accountability and saw no reason to make an exception when it came to medical professionals. Thus after the Coalition won the NSW parliamentary election in 1988, they never threatened the existence of the CU in any way but rather willingly supported its continued existence.

Still, by the end of the 1980s, NSW had fallen behind other Australian jurisdictions, since all had established their health complaints bodies as full-blown statutory authorities. In contrast, the CU continued to be a mere departmental unit, subject to the whims of a minister who had the power at any time to terminate its operations. An independent statutory authority would not be subject to any such threat, but when moves began to advance the CU to that status, they were met with furious opposition by several surprising opponents because these were consumerist organisations.

Chief among them was a body called the Medical Consumers' Association, the views of which were supported not only by the *Sun Herald* newspaper but also by formidable rightwing political commentators such as Alan Jones, whose daily tirades on the 2GB radio station were and still are carefully noted by governments of the day. Jones lined up behind the demands of the Medical Consumers' Association that the chief purpose of the CU should be to obtain financial compensation for those who had suffered injury and harm in the course of medical treatment.[9] The CU rejected this view, arguing that such an approach would be costly and complex and do little to expose systemic shortcomings in State's health care provision which was seen to be the underlying purpose of the CU. On the grounds that individual injury was indicative of systemic pathology, the leaders of the CU held the view that systemic reform was more important than individual redress.[10] On their part NSW governments, ever resistant to the prospect of large new and unproductive expenditures which would result from any agreement to pay compensation to those who had suffered injury during their medical treatment, supported this position.

Given these differences of opinion, it is not surprising that when a bill to upgrade the status of the CU to that of a statutory authority was introduced in the NSW Parliament in 1991, it gave rise to fierce debate and contest both outside and inside the Parliament. That the bill finally passed was due to two factors. The first was the support of the Coalition Government of the day, which demonstrates the crucial importance of its ideological shift described earlier. However, the Coalition had been almost fatally weakened by the most recent State election and continued to occupy the government benches only with the support of four independents in the Lower House. By itself it probably would have lacked the nerve to pass the Act transforming the CU into a statutory authority

However, its backbone was strengthened by the herculean lobbying efforts of the Public Interest Advocacy Centre, an activist group based in the legal profession. They were opposed to the idea of financial compensation for the victims of medical malpractice on the same grounds as the CU. With that extra-parliamentary encouragement, the Coalition government, on the basis of the thinnest of margins viz the Speaker's casting vote in the Lower House, managed to pass the Health Care Complaints Commission Act at the end of 1993.[11] That was a momentous development; but as we shall see, it was to give rise to a totally unanticipated regulatory development affecting the practice of UCM.

UCM drawn into the medical accountability net

In 1986, two years after her appointment to the Complaints Unit (CU), Smith resigned and was succeeded by Ms (now Professor Dr) Merrilyn Walton whose activist background was in the legal aid movement. Under her leadership, the CU moved in important new directions, one of the most significant, in line with recommendations of the Chelmsford Hospital Royal Commission, was the upgrading of its status to that of a statutory authority.

When it became such, the name of the CU changed to that of the Health Care Complaints Commission (HCCC from this point onwards). What was to prove as significant if not an even more momentous change, was that its investigatory powers, which up until then had been confined to governmental health care institutions, were now widened to include complaints against individual health professionals and organisations in the private sector. Yet among the HCCC's new powers which were to prove most significant from the point of view of this study was, as recorded in its 1996 Annual Report, a little noticed statement that it had been empowered to deal with complaints against 'other types of health care providers'. The reference here was to practitioners of UCM, something which reflected the fact that as reported by Walton, the HCCC had been receiving complaints made by disgruntled clients of such practitioners.

That this was the case was confirmed in the first report submitted to the NSW Legislative Assembly by its 'Committee on the Health Care Complaints Commission' established in terms of the 1993 Act which had brought the HCCC into existence. This committee, composed of Members of both houses of Parliament, was tasked with holding regular meetings with the directorate of the HCCC and reporting back to the Parliament on an annual basis. Significantly, in its first report issued in 1998, this Committee stated it had given special consideration to '...the adequacy and appropriateness of current mechanisms for resolving complaints against unregistered health practitioners' because of

> ...repeated comments by the Commissioner about the HCCC's limited ability to protect the public from unprofessional treatment given by unregistered health practitioners.[12]

The 'unregistered health practitioners' were of course, those practising UCM. Dealing with them posed a major difficulty:

neither the Complaints Unit nor later the HCCC had ever been empowered to take direct punitive action against practitioners they had found to be guilty of professional misconduct. Instead as already related, they had to refer such cases to one of the 14 statutory health professional registration bodies such as the Medical Registration Board which alone had the power to refer miscreant and erring practitioners to the Medical Tribunal.

As governments had no doubt believed long before Sheehan made his seminal statement of 1956, any law which sought to control UCM practice would also need to be enforced by professional registration boards. However, as we have seen in the previous chapter, apart from chiropractic and osteopathy (and in Victoria, Traditional Chinese Medicine), governments had refused to bestow similar professional registration powers on any UCM modalities or on their practitioners.

In consequence, as recorded by the Parliamentary Committee, while many groups within the UCM field had put in place self-regulatory mechanisms, their effectiveness relied on the 'goodwill and responsibility' of individuals. But that was often lacking among practitioners and noted the Committee, self-regulation was 'a voluntary process' and that 'numerous unregistered health practitioners legitimately chose not to be governed by even this level of regulation.' Moreover, 'it would appear that the range of mechanisms available to complain about unregistered health practitioners only provided very limited and piecemeal protection for health consumers'.[13]

To emphasise that point, the Committee report further set out in detail the way some customers of UCM practitioners had been defrauded and the failure of treatments provided by practitioners. Their lack of anything like medical registers in UCM organisations from which miscreant practitioners could be 'struck off', meant they had no power to control or discipline their members and thus it was futile to refer complaints to them.

The Half-Grail of 'negative regulation'

Finding a way of dealing with such complaints was anything but easy. That this regulatory Grail proved to be almost as elusive as the original Grail is evidenced by the fact that ten years after its establishment, the expenditure of many hours in discussion, the production of many substantial reports and the making of multiple recommendations such as that 'professional [UCM] associations ... put in complaint mechanisms and adopt disciplinary processes like the registration boards' (which for reasons cited earlier, turned out to be impracticable), the HCCC Parliamentary Committee noted in its 2004 report that there was still 'real cause for concern about the lack of regulation of unregistered practitioners and the consequent inability for them to be sanctioned for unprofessional behaviour'.[14]

But in fact a first step towards moving around this disciplinary cul-de-sac had been suggested by the Parliamentary Committee in a major report on *The Adequacy and Appropriateness of Current Mechanisms for Resolving Complaints* presented to the NSW Parliament in 1998. That report proposed the adoption of 'a more generic form of registration for all alternative health practitioners'. Such a system, it was suggested, could be made operable by the passing of 'an umbrella type of legislation which would capture alternative practitioners under ... generic disciplinary procedures'.[15]

This recommendation was repeated in another Committee document on the *History and Roles of the Committee on the Health Care Complaints Commission, 1994-2004* which again raised the question of how to take action against miscreant UCM practitioners. Although as noted earlier, these were being reported to the HCCC, the only weak action the HCCC could take was to send 'adverse comments' to such practitioners, who mostly ignored them. Still, no doubt bearing in mind that this was an era of when de-regulation (as embodied in the recommendations of the Hilmer Report of 1998) was very much in vogue, the Committee also stated that it did not 'necessarily support the view that professional registration of these [i.e. UCM] professions is the answer'.[16]

An early step towards dealing with this regulatory dilemma had been suggested by this same Committee as early as 1996 when it cited, as noted above, the 'umbrella' model of regulation adopted in the Canadian province of Ontario, as a way forward. That model was based on the novel concept of 'negative regulation'.[13] This concept can best be understood by comparing it to orthodox regulation, in terms of which governments legislate to ensure that only those with requisite qualifications (mostly those issued by tertiary institutions) are allowed to practice in a particular field. In the case of medical practice, as related in Chapter 1 at the outset in NSW these included only those with qualifications from the ancient British universities.

That of course was in time expanded to include all universities with medical training faculties, the first of which in Australia was the University of Sydney. The operation of the regulatory system was and is placed in the hands of a controlling body which in the medical field in NSW was the Medical Board first set up in 1838, but armed with regulatory 'teeth' only after 1901. As noted in Chapter 1, that body (which later became the Medical Registration Board) was also made responsible for maintaining a register of those it deemed qualified to practice in that field.

From 1938, this body was also tasked with enforcing discipline by taking action against practitioners who failed to meet the required standards of practice, being empowered to receive and consider any such cases and after 1987, if it found them deserving of further action, referring such cases to a Medical Tribunal. Operating in terms of the procedures of a court of law, that body makes final judgements on the fitness of the accused practitioner to continue to practice, and orders anyone adjudged to be unfit of practice to be 'struck off the roll' i.e. the Medical Register.

In contrast to this rather complicated system, in terms of negative regulation no qualifications are required of anyone wanting to practice in any particular field. This may have seemed like a reversion to the 'free-for-all' pre-1900 situation described in

Chapters 1 and 2. However, in terms of negative regulation, anyone who practices UCM is bound by law to comply with a legislated Code of Conduct. Such a Code requires practitioners among other things, to provide services in a safe and ethical manner, never to practice under the influence of alcohol or drugs, never to claim the ability to cure serious diseases such as cancer, not financially to exploit clients, to keep appropriate records and have adequate and appropriate insurance. All UCM practitioners are required to display the Code in their workplace where it can easily be seen by their clientele. (The full NSW Code appears in Appendix 2). Any client who believes that a practitioner has violated any aspect of the Code, has the right to complain to a governmental instrumentality empowered to take action against that practitioner.

Finding such an instrumentality however, proved to be anything but easy for the HCCC Parliamentary Committee which was tasked with this problem. In its report of 1998 the that Committee recorded that there were a number of laws and instrumentalities which aggrieved UCM clients could use for the satisfaction or any complaints they may have had. However, the Committee concluded:

> It would appear that the range of mechanisms available to complain about unregistered health practitioners only provide very limited and piecemeal protection for health consumers. Further, many of the agencies who administer the relevant Acts do not see the protection of standards of health care as their core business.[17]

Eventually in 2006 (twelve years after it began to consider the issue) the Committee came to a conclusion which in retrospect, seems obvious: that the agency best equipped not only to deal with complaints about UCM practitioners but also to take punitive action against them, was the Health Care Complaints Commission (HCCC). Its acceptance of that fact of life was embodied in the formal words of its report, in which the Committee recommended that the HCCC be 'given the power to determine that a health practitioner has breached the code of conduct ...' [18] That would solve the problem of how complaints against UCM practitioners could be investigated. But the Committee went much further when it recommended that that if the HCCC found a practitioner guilty of violating any aspect of the Code of Conduct, it be empowered 'to make a prohibition order restricting all or certain aspects their practice or for a specified period of time'. [18] That meant that the HCCC had been equipped with punitive powers similar to those of the Medical Tribunal.

When these recommendations were accepted and given legal force by the Unregistered Practitioners Act of 2006 (later replaced by the Public Health Act of 2010) that introduced a new medical regulatory regime. That regime 'short-circuited' as it were, the existing complaints system by giving the HCCC the power not only to investigate complaints against UCM practitioners, but also to take disciplinary action against them. The new system was accepted with little debate in either House of the NSW Parliament and given legislative force in the form of the Public Health Regulation Act of 2010.

The radical outcome of this new system was that anyone practising any kind of health or vaguely health-related modality, was now free to operate in NSW. These included practitioners of acupuncture, audiology, dietitians, counselling, herbalism, homeopathy, dental technicians, hypnotherapy, massage therapy, occupational therapy, naturopathy, phlebotomy, radiography, reiki and speech therapy and also practitioners offering cosmetic facial and physical enhancement.

While it may seem that in terms of negative regulation all UCM modalities were being allowed to practice without let or hindrance, in fact they were now obliged to work under a regulatory regime governed by the Code of Conduct which by law, had to be prominently displayed in practitioners' consulting rooms (the NSW version is fully reproduced in Appendix 2). That Code was and is 'policed' by their customers who, if they believe they had been harmed or defrauded by a practitioner of any UCM modality or provider of cosmetic services, could take their complaints to the HCCC with its new powers to investigate and take punitive action against practitioners complained about. Examples of this system in operation appear in Appendix 3.

When the Act came into force in 2012, the same year that the Australian Health Practitioners Authority (AHPRA) commenced its operations, it betokened that for the first time in the post-invasion/settlement history of NSW, the practice of UCM had been brought within the regulatory purview of the S[s]tate. That, for the State itself, was a huge regulatory step forward. What is historically significant about negative regulation is that working through the Parliamentary Committee, it was the HCCC, rooted as it was in the seemingly obscure field of health complaints, that had proved to be the most eager seeker and eventual finder of this particular regulatory prize.

At this point it can be noted that after an extensive Australia-wide consultation process, the Commonwealth Health Ministers Advisory Council reported in 2013 that there was general agreement that the NSW model provided the most effective regulatory mechanism for disciplining erring and miscreant UCM practitioners. As a result, most Australian jurisdictions have to date adopted or are in the process of adopting that model.

Another significant aspect of the 2010 legislation in NSW was the way in which it expanded the scope of HCCC activities. Most notably, in terms of Section 7 of the Act, the Commission was empowered to investigate complaints against beauty therapists and cosmetic modification technicians and also complaints made about organisations such as cosmetic and beauty clinics.[19] What this meant was the scope of HCCC investigations had moved beyond the purely health complaints sphere into that of public health, because what was becoming clear was that the burgeoning and uncontrolled cosmetic enhancement industry had the potential to cause serious harm to its clientele. Just how serious was made tragically clear in 2017 when the owner of a beauty salon who was undergoing a breast enhancement procedure by a visiting friend, died after being administered the wrong anaesthetics.

Negative regulation in practice

Whatever the shortcomings of negative regulation, one major benefit was that it brought UCM into the statistical purview of the HCCC. What has emerged from that development is that the number of complaints against UCM practitioners is miniscule over against those against registered practitioners and medical institutions, amounting to only 2-3% of the total number of health complaints annually. Successive HCCC annual reports show that while the number of complaints against MM practitioners have risen steadily reaching 1,224 in 2016-17, between 2010 and that date there were only 52 complaints against UCM practitioners. Moreover the numbers of complaints against the latter have remained largely static year-on-year, while a good number of these have concerned not practice issues but 'boundary violations', which involve practitioners making unwanted sexual advances to their clients.

The reasons for the low numbers of complaints about UCM practice and practitioners reported to the HCCC are not clear. It could be that the existence of the HCCC's investigatory powers is simply unknown to the great mass of the users of UCM, or that a great number of such users distrust governmental bodies. It could also be that cases of malpractice and malfeasance among UCM practitioners are comparatively rare; that may be due to the generally non-invasive nature of UCM practice causing only a very low number of physical or mental harm to its clientele. Whatever the reason, the HCCC reports indicate that charges by some MM protagonists that UCM is 'dangerous', are not supported by the statistics. On that score, negative regulation has handed UCM if not a victory in its 'war' with MM, then at least a useful debating point.

It should be remarked here that after an extensive Australia-wide consultation process, the Health Ministers Advisory Council reported in 2013 that there was general agreement that the NSW model provided the most effective regulatory mechanism for disciplining erring and miscreant UCM practitioners.

The pros and cons of negative regulation

Negative regulation has not been without its critics among UCM protagonists. Foremost among them is Dr Jon Wardle at the University of Technology Sydney and editor of the journal *Advances in Integrative Medicine*. He has argued that since Codes of Conduct do not establish standards which need to be met by those wishing to practise a UCM modality, they do not ensure that practitioners have high levels of skill and knowledge either before or during the course of their practice. They therefore 'do not offer much preventive protection through the promotion of higher standards of training or practice.'[20]

Wardle was correct in pointing out that this meant that negative regulation falls short of being the full Grail of professional registration. He and others, including Dr Kerryn Phelps who, as we have seen, served three-year presidential terms of both the AMA and AIMA, continue to argue for the granting of full professional registration status to UCM modalities. That would make them, along with chiropractic, osteopathy and Traditional Chinese medicine, not only participants in the national AHPRA medical regulatory organisation, but would also signal that UCM had at last gained full governmental and therefore societal recognition.

Among the voices of those demanding full professional registration for UCM modalities is that of the Australian Natural Therapists' Association which claims to represent 'the multi-disciplinary interests of approximately 10,500 accredited practitioners Australia-wide'. That body continues to

> '...lobby the government and government departments to include Naturopaths, Homeopaths, Herbalists (Western), Nutritionists, Musculoskeletal Therapists,

Myotherapists, Remedial Therapists, Shiatsu Therapists, Aromatherapists and Ayurvedic Medicine Practitioners to be registered under the National Registration and Accreditation Scheme.[21]

However, the governments involved in the AHPRA are unlikely quickly to fulfil that aspiration. For one thing, there is continued resistance to the creation of more health bureaucracies dating back to the Hilmer report of 1998. And no doubt in both Commonwealth and State spheres, there is likely to be a lively consciousness of the ongoing fierce critiques of UCM by bodies such as the Friends of Science in Medicine described in the next chapter and also hostile media outlets. Granting full registration to the plethora of UCM modalities listed in the statement of the Australian Natural Therapies Association statement would provoke as much political uproar as any attempt to suppress them. And as confirmed by Minister Sheehan in his seminal statement of 1956, that kind of uproar is something governments studiously try to avoid.

CHAPTER 9

The Conflict Continues

While Mainstream Medicine (MM) is the officially recognised and supported system of health care In NSW and Australia as a whole, it should be clear from earlier chapters that this does not imply any wholesale rejection of UnConventional Medicine (UCM) by governments. The attitude of the NSW government was conveyed to the author by an official in the Health Department who stated that while 'NSW Health does not employ complementary or alternative therapists', it did make plentiful information about UCM available on the Departmental website and that similar information could be found on the website of the NSW Agency for Clinical Innovation.[2] Which leads to the conclusion that the current official attitude of the NSW government to UCM is the same as that of NHMRC quoted earlier: 'Acknowledge, but don't encourage'.

This approach could lead to the conclusion that while much had changed in governmental attitudes towards UCM since the late 20th century, in fact at a basic level, little or nothing had changed since Sheahan made his seminal statement in 1956. The advances made by UCM in popular acceptance and in the media and academic spheres have not betokened any major rolling back MM's control of the commanding heights of the health care system in NSW, particularly the hospital and public health sectors. Thus, despite the growing legitimacy of UCM, MM remained the dominant paradigm in the health care field. If as the Expert Committee's report suggested in 2006, UCM had been recognised as a playing a significant role in the maintenance of good population health in NSW, an overall assessment of the situation indicates that not only in the eyes of the State government but also those of the media, it is still very much a junior role.

A telling indication of that was furnished in October 2018 by a parliamentary by-election in the 'up-market' Sydney seat of Wentworth. That seat had been held by the conservative parties for 117 years until its incumbent Mr Malcolm Turner, who had been Prime Minister of Australia, was voted out of its leadership by his party. In consequence he resigned as the MP for Wentworth. When the by-election to fill the vacancy took place, it was sensationally won by Dr Kerryn Phelps standing as an independent. Her earlier embrace of UCM and elevation to the leadership of the Australian Integrative Medicine Association (AIMA) has been outlined in Chapter 6.

Yet while she was the focus of huge attention from both local and foreign media both during and after during the by-election campaign and her 2002-05 presidency of the AMA received constant mention, nowhere did her three-year (2009-2012) presidential term of the Australasian Integrative Medicine Association (AIMA) receive any mention at all. That indicates that despite its widespread usage, UCM remains a somewhat obscure presence in the overall health system of NSW and of Australia as a whole.

Moreover, its right to play any role in that system continued to be challenged in the 21st century by organisations such as the Australian Skeptics who, in their magazine *The Skeptic,* have kept up a drumfire of criticism and rejection of UCM because of its apparently non-scientific nature. In 2017 the Skeptics bestowed their 'Bent Spoon' award, given each year to individuals or organisations which in the Skeptics' view, have claimed fantastical results for unprovable paranormal activities. In 2017 the 'Bent Spoon' was awarded to the National Institute of Complementary Medicine (NICM) on the grounds that it was '… continuing to fully support and defend the use of homeopathy and other unbelievable complementary medicines [and] ignoring the detrimental impact that their approach have on science, scientific education and the general health and wellbeing of the Australian population.' When the award was officially announced, the Skeptics accused the NICM of

> ... promoting unproven treatments and now also [being] involved in a project to establish a clinic for Traditional Chinese Medicine on the campus of the University of Western Sydney. The 2017 winner's involvement is described as 'clinical trials', but the University acknowledges that the TCM clinic may be opened to the public – a highly dubious pseudomedicine given the imprimatur of university "research". [3]

Similar critiques were also visible in both tabloid print media such as *The Sunday Telegraph*, the deputy-editor of which, Claire Harvey in 2016 authored an editorial entitled 'Don't duck the law by taking kids to quacks.' Among other things, she wrote:

> ... let's be honest, [N]aturopaths are quacks. So are chiropractors, traditional Chinese herbalists, iridologists, palm-readers, homeopaths, Bowen therapists and reiki practitioners. Quack, quack, quack. ... And if you fall for their nonsense I think you deserve exactly what you get. That is, nothing.[4]

In the more academic online publication *The Conversation*, UCM also came under critical scrutiny from legal/academic quarters[5, 6,7] the Melbourne-based *Journal of Law and Medicine* being highly critical of homeopathy in particular.[8]

A new and formidable opponent of UCM emerged in 2011 when it began to be vigorously attacked by a body calling itself 'Friends of Science in Medicine' (FSM) under the leadership of Emeritus Professor John Dwyer of the Medical Faculty of the University of New South Wales which set as a primary goal the elimination of the teaching of UCM courses in tertiary institutions. In January 2015, Dr Dwyer announced that FSM had already attracted 1,000 members, double its membership in 2012, most of these being drawn from the academic sphere.

Typical of the attacks on UCM in the FSM's newsletters, was one which asserted that:

> Complementary and alternative medicines' (CAMs) are the modern version of magical practices. They are mostly ineffective. At their worst, they are dangerous…

This article further argued that

> The teaching of so-called health courses or topics such as homeopathy, reflexology, chiropractic, iridology etc. in our universities and other tertiary institutions … contradicts the commitment of these institutions to maintaining the highest educational and research standards, compromises the real science taught in those institutions and gives undue credibility to unscientific practices: our healthcare system should not tolerate these so-called professions with their roots in non-scientific principles.[9]

In early 2019 the Friends of Science appeared to have won a significant victory when the University of Technology Sydney (UTS) announced it was closing the degree course in Traditional Chinese Medicine which, as we have seen, was the first UCM course to be established at any university in New South Wales. The closure move was on the grounds that the course was no longer financially viable and did not produce enough research. Justifying the decision, one of FSM's leaders, Associate Professor Ken Harvey of the School of Public Health and Preventive Medicine at Monash University, asserted that there was little to back up the therapeutic claims of TCM which pre-dated the scientific era. However a spokesman for the UTS said that the debate over the scientific validity of TCM had nothing to do with the decision and was 'in no way a reflection of an institutional bias against complementary health care'.[10]

Earlier in 2019 however, UCM had scored a victory of its own when a Commonwealth governmental ban on Medicare rebates for a long list of UCM treatments recommended by the then Chief Commonwealth Medical Officer Professor Chris Baggoley, who in 2013 had found there was no clear evidence supporting any of the therapies. However, when the Commonwealth Department of Health proposed acting on his recommendation in 2019, that was challenged by a vocal campaign staged by practitioners and users of UCM, who sent over 13,000 protests to the Commonwealth government Minister of Health Mr Greg Hunt. Among the protesters was Dr Kerryn Phelps who at that time was still an MP and who personally approached the Minister urging him to lift the rebate restriction on several of the therapies. She told him that 'Australians are continuing to turn to natural therapies,' and that there was clear evidence that 'there could be savings in public expenditure if complementary medicines were better supported by private health insurance'. The Minister accepted her arguments and ordered a review of the withdrawal of rebates on five therapies a week after they had been introduced.[11]

Apart from its victory in the case of the closure of the Traditional Chinese Medicine course at the University of Technology, to date the Friends of Science organisation has not made much progress in its campaigns against UCM, one reason being that mentioned in the previous chapter – that as a result of its inroads into the academic sphere, UCM is itself now supported by a significant cohort of academics. Thus, in response to the FSM demand that the teaching of UCM courses be eliminated from the universities, a group of such academics (who included Dr Kerryn Phelps) wrote in an editorial in the *Medical Journal of Australia* that while they agreed 'that any university degrees in complementary medicine should have a strong foundation in the biomedical sciences', they none the less argued: 'Science does not occur in a vacuum; it is a social phenomenon, a practice that is embedded in the wider cultural values and power relationships in society.' That meant that if the FSM were to succeed in its stated aims, 'they would achieve a dystopia – a medical "1984" - where only one way of knowing the body in health and illness is permitted in public discourse.'[12]

Something of a truce between the proponents of the FSM and those of UCM was called when in 2018, the head of the NICM Dr Alan Bensoussan, invited the FSM's Dr John Dwyer and another notable critic of UCM, Associate Professor Ken Harvey mentioned earlier, to visit the headquarters of the NICM at the University of Western Sydney to meet its staff and inspect its laboratories. This face-to-face encounter between the chief opponents in the 'war' did not result in any hostile confrontations and afterwards Dr Dwyer told the author that he was impressed by the standards of equipment in the NICM laboratories. While the encounter did not result in any reconciliation either, Dr Bensoussan states that he afterwards detected a slight softening of the attacks on UCM by Drs Dwyer and Harvey.

The existence of Friends of Science and its arguments forcefully and continuously set out on its website, together with the hostility to UCM in various media and academic bodies mentioned earlier, doubtless stands as a warning to governments. Clearly, showing too much favour to UCM by for instance, heeding the pleas for greater research funding and the extension of full registration to UCM modalities could, as noted in the previous chapter, create politically dangerous furores.

Avoiding such furores means that governments keep their options open in a contest in which neither MM or UCM has been able to score a decisive victory. While as a result of spectacular medical advance over the last century MM dominates the health field, its failures evident for instance in the critiques of and hostility towards the medical profession and MM generally, which led to the formation of the NSW Complaints Unit in 1985 and after 2000, to the growth of the Health Care Complaints Commission and similar bodies throughout Australia and also overseas, has meant that it has never been able to establish total control of the field. And that, as has been demonstrated in earlier chapters, has also been due to sociological forces such as post-modernism and economic forces such as consumerism. Even more decisive have been the political developments under both Labor and Liberal governments which led as already mentioned, to the formation of the CU and the HCCC.

Yet while the fortunes of UCM have benefited from these developments and it gained a greater following and degree of recognition in the late 20th century, the great bulk of UCM modalities have never attained, as already argued, more than a junior status in the health field. Thus UCM modalities such as naturopathy have made little progress in their quest for the Holy Grail of official regulation attained by the MM (and some UCM) modalities which fall within the purview of the Australasian Health Practitioners Regulatory Authority (AHPRA). At the same time the degree of following and support for UCM evident throughout the history of NSW, make governments in both the Commonwealth and State spheres, Sheahan-like to be wary of taking action against it as they have been urged to do by organisations such as the Skeptics and Friends of Science in Medicine.

Thus the two health universes of thinking and practice embodied in the contending forces of MM and UCM continue to contend and conflict in a 'war' which as set out in this work, dates back to the beginning of the existence of modern New South Wales 200 years ago and of course long before that. The conflict over medical practice in NSW is just a microcosm of that not only in Australia but in the whole of the economically developed largely Western world over a millennium.

For their part, contemporary governments of whatever ideological persuasion, sceptical as they tend to be of UCM' therapeutic claims, are also uneasily aware of the probable electoral consequences of showing too much favour or disfavour to either side. Thus they tend not to attempt to play any greater role than that of a reluctant referee. Sometimes the governmental referee makes some surprising decisions. Thus in May 2018, the Commonwealth government accepted only three of 45 recommendations of a high-level Pharmacy Remuneration and Regulation Panel, merely noting but failing to act on the 30 other recommendations from this Panel designed to restrict the sale of complementary medicines in pharmacies, particularly including homeopathic remedies.[13]

'Aluta continua' – the struggle continues.

Of course, the war between MM and UCM has also raged in other States and Territories and in the Commonwealth sphere. In fact, a major battle that is being fought out as the final Chapter of this book is being written. Although that battle is being fought out in the Commonwealth sphere, it is worth describing and analysing it as far as possible because it encapsulates all the elements of the war in NSW. The opening shots were heard in early 2019 when the Commonwealth Medical Board of Australia operating under the aegis of the AHPRA, issued a major public consultation paper on 'clearer regulation of medical practitioners who provide complementary and unconventional medicine and emerging treatments'. In its long justification for its investigation this Board noted several times that the use of UCM was increasing and that while it did not 'wish to stifle or limit the rights of patients to choose their healthcare' … it felt there was a need for 'additional safeguards to protect patients who sought such treatments'.

The goal of this exercise was set out in the form of two options, the first being to leave intact the existing status quo under which the Board had no interaction with UCM modalities, the second to 'strengthen current guidelines for medical practitioners who provide complementary and unconventional medicine through practice-specific guidelines that clearly articulate the Board's expectations of all medical practitioners …' The Board stated its preference to be this second option.[14]

Here we need to pause and compare this new phase of the struggle between MM and UCM with those of earlier eras. In the 19th century, as outlined in Chapters 1-3, the demand of the leaders in the MM camp in NSW was that governments 'put down quackery', in other words, eliminate its practice by legal means. Having experienced the power of UCM in both the NSW parliament and outside, State governments never made any move to comply with this demand.

A major reason for that was supplied by Health Minister Sheahan in 1956 when he implied that governments thought it best to regard UCM as a sleeping dog which could be left to lie undisturbed somewhere in *terra incognita*. Over the next five decades, as described in Chapter 6, UCM proved that it was anything but asleep and moreover its territory was thoroughly mapped by both its leaders and the NSW government. But individuals who had had negative experiences with UCM practitioners and also governments as embodied particularly in the Health Care Complaints Commission (HCCC), still hankered after some sort of control UCM. That aim was finally achieved in the form of the Act of 2010 which implemented the concept of 'negative regulation', the NSW lead being followed by most other States and Territories in Australia.

In 2019 the Commonwealth Medical Board made no reference whatsoever to this existing regulatory regime in its position paper. Still, that paper embodied a new phase in the war in that while it did not attack UCM in any way, it set out as delineated above, the Board's aim of subjecting UCM practitioners to the same controls as those applying to MM practitioners. In other words, while the Medical Board was not aiming to suppress UCM in any way, it was moving to control UCM practice.

But while the tone of the Board's position paper was conciliatory and did not evidence any 'put-down-quackery' mindset, it provoked a huge negative response from the UCM camp, most notably in the form of over 11,000 submissions from organisations and individual users of UCM therapies strongly opposed to any move by the Board to exercise any kind of control over UCM practitioners. That this proposed action was interpreted by many as indeed a move to 'put-down-quackery' is indicated by the fact that a large number of individual submissions detailed how UCM therapies had helped and in many cases, healed the authors of the submissions. In other words, even without formal qualifications or recognition, UCM practitioners were seen by the great majority of their clientele to be effective and not in need of any official permission to practice.

Foremost among the organisational responses from NSW was that of the National Institute of Complementary Medicine (NICM) which among other things stated flatly that 'no additional regulation of doctors who use complementary medicine is required'. Another NSW response came from Professor Stephen Myers of the Southern Cross University, a leading proponent of UCM, who asserted that what was being proposed by the Medical Board 'smacks to me of a situation where we want not only to suppress these people [i.e. the practitioners of UCM] ... but we want to make sure they can't talk, they can't research, they can't advise, they can't engage in policy development.'[11]

The time which the Medical Board will need to complete the process and respond to the flood of submissions, places its findings and proposals outside the timeframe of this book. Whatever its findings, its investigation also makes it clear that after their two centuries of strife, the 'war' between MM and UCM in both the State or Commonwealth spheres is not likely to end any time soon.

Conclusion – the power of non-medical factors

That if as argued earlier, governments have and still do play that 'referee' role in that 'war' is one more indication that, as argued throughout this work, it is political factors along with socio/economic factors rather than solely or merely medical factors, that have played major roles in determining the state of the contest between MM and UCM in NSW and in the world outside its borders.

Thus, as outlined in the opening chapters of this work, in the 19th century it was economically-based class factors as much as the efficacy of their competing medical epistemologies which determined the strength of the respective followings of UCM and MM. The increasing medical expertise and efficacy of MM in the early to mid-20th century elevated it to being the dominant paradigm of health care and re-inforced its recognition and acceptance by governments. That in turn eroded the class basis of the UCM's following and led to its political eclipse in NSW in 1938. But the social failings of the medical profession such as the NSW Medical Registration Board's abuse of power outlined in Chapter 5, led to a rising volume of critiques of MM which in turn eroded its power and also its following not only among the members of the public, but also within the medical profession itself. That was evident for instance, the in the formation of the Doctors' Reform Society in 1973 and the Australasian Integrative Medicine Association in 1992.

The resulting decline in the profession's social standing coupled with the effect of factors such as the rise of consumerism and the advent of social movements, particularly the non-authoritarian philosophy of post-modernism as outlined in Chapter 6, enabled UCM to surge back into public consciousness and usage and also gain greater governmental acknowledgement in the later 20th and early 21st centuries. Acknowledgement did not imply official recognition however, and as noted earlier in this chapter, apart from chiropractic, osteopathy and Traditional Chinese Medicine, none of the plethora of UCM modalities has been able to attain the Holy Grail of government regulation which they are still earnestly seeking but which governments are reluctant and, perhaps nervously unwilling to grant.

It might be remarked that in the ongoing 'war', those critics of UCM such as the FSM and journalist Claire Harvey quoted earlier, have continued to argue against and condemn UCM on purely medical/scientific grounds without taking into account the socio/political factors outlined in this work. Moreover, strong critics of UCM such as the Skeptics and the Friends of Science either pay no heed to or are ignorant of recent research into UCM usage by the general population such as that carried out by McIntyre *et al.* In their survey of complementary medicine use by a 'broadly representative' sample of 2,019 members of the Australian population aged 18 years and over, they found that

> The prevalence of consultations with either a naturopath or Western herbalist has remained steady over the past decade. However, this study found younger adults were more likely to consult with naturopaths and Western herbalists, in contrast with literature reporting higher rates of [UCM] use in middle-aged Australians … The stable use of complementary medicine in the Australian population in general, and naturopathy in particular, may be contributing to a normalisation of these historically "alternative" medicines.[15]

Two points arise from this conclusion. Firstly, as delineated in this book, the use of UCM in NSW anyway (and very probably in the rest of Australia), has been 'normalised' among a good segment population not only contemporaneously, but for the past 200 years. Secondly, the finding that 'younger adults' were more likely to consult with naturopaths and Western herbalists, indicates that UCM is no danger of dying out due the ageing of its clientele.

This point was already clear from the 2018 survey of Steel *et al* who found that fully 63% of the 2019 individuals 'broadly representative of the Australian population' who were surveyed, were between the ages of 18 and 39. They concluded that 'prevalence of [U]CM use in Australia has remained consistently high, demonstrating that [U]CM is an established part of contemporary health management practices within the general population'.[16] Again, in the light of what has been said earlier, it should be added that UCM's role in 'contemporary health management' practices is a very junior one.

Not that every aspect of MM's role has been spectacularly successful. While the use of scientific methodologies has enabled MM to make huge and spectacular advances in the understanding and treatment of ill-health, it has none the less failed to make much progress or none at all to date in understanding the causes of let alone defeating many deadly diseases such as pancreatic cancer. That would indicate that there are still large areas of related to health which scientific methodologies have yet to explain.

One idea that has been put forward is that UCM works largely and perhaps solely through the placebo effect. But even if that is true, it hardly advances any scientific explanation of how UCM therapies work because to date there has been no scientific explanation of how the placebo effect itself works. Moreover, that as detailed in Chapter 1, no scientific basis has been discovered for the widely used practice of acupuncture, challenges any idea that only 'scientifically-based' therapies should be used when treating infirmity and disease.

Perhaps the most telling challenge to that idea lies in the field of anaesthetics. These have been hugely improved and well-nigh universally used since their discovery close on 200 years ago.[17] Yet while, as any simple internet search will demonstrate, the subject of anaesthetics has attracted a huge amount of research and an equally huge amount of literature and ongoing study, there is still no scientific understanding of how or why anaesthics work.[18] That gap in the knowledge-base of medical science has never been seen as any reason to refuse the use of anaesthetics. The same could be true of many UCM therapies.

It might be said that this work has attempted to adopt a neutral stance in the war between MM and UCM, the author seeing himself as neither an opponent or proponent of UCM. He first became aware of the ongoing 'war' between them when he was researching for his doctorate in the records of the 19th century NSW Parliament. His surprise at the ferocity of the conflict there was the greater because he was aware of the equally ferocious clashes between elements of MM and UCM in the 21st century. His curiosity about the reasons for long lasting nature of the two-century long 'war' between them, opened a wide field of research he was able to delve into after he retired from teaching in the School of Public

Health and Community Medicine in the University of New South Wales – although it should be said that that University and its Medicine Faculty generally pay little or no attention to UCM! However, without the generous and academically impartial way in which the School and the University made their research facilities and resources available to the author, the writing of this account of would not have been possible.

In conclusion, it should be recorded that *Two Hundred Years of Strife* has been compiled not only to fill a gap in the historical record of New South Wales, but also in the hope that the 'health wars' both in this geo-political 'laboratory' and also in the world beyond, can be better understood.

NOTES

CHAPTER 1 - *REFERENCES*

1. New South Wales Legislative Council. Act to define the qualifications of Medical Witnesses at Coroners' Inquests and Inquiries held before Justices of the Peace in the Colony of NSW (2 Victoria 22). 1838.

2. New South Wales. Report from the Committee on the Medical Practice Bill with the minutes of evidence. Sydney: The Legislative Council; 1838.

3. ibid.

4. Porter R. *Health for Sale; Quackery in England, 1660-1850.* Manchester: Manchester University Press; 1989.

5. Martyr P. *Paradise of Quacks.* Sydney: Macleay Press; 2002.

6. National Health and Medical Research Council (NHMRC). Official Statement on Homeopathy. 2015.

7. O'Neill A, Willis, E. Chiropractic and the politics of health care. *Australian Journal of Public Health.* 1994; 18:325-31.

8. Zhu X, Carlton A, Bensoussan A. Development and change for traditional Chinese medicine in Australia. *The Journal of Alternative and Complementary Medicine.* 2009; 15:685-8.

9. Litscher G. No, there is no conclusive scientific evidence of visualisatioons of meridians at the moment. *The Journal of Alternative and Complementary Medicine.* 2014; 20:215-6.

10. Lloyd P. *A social history of medicine; medical professionalisation in New South Wales, 1788-1950.* [Doctoral]. Sydney: University of New South Wales; 1993.

11. Willis E. *Medical dominance; the division of labour in Australian health care.* Sydney: Allen & Unwin; 1991.

12. Wannan W. *Folk medicine; a miscellany of old cures and remedies,*

superstitions, and old wives' tales having particular reference to Australia and the British Isles. Melbourne: Hill of Content; 1970.

13. New South Wales. *The wealth and progress of New South Wales.* Sydney: W.A. Gulick Government Printer; 1902.

14. Bruck L. *The Australasian medical directory and hand-book* Sydney: Australian Medical Gazette; 1883.

15. Pensabene T. *The rise of the medical practitioner in Victoria.* Canberra: Australian National University; 1980.

16. New South Wales. Parliamentary Debates 1887(a), p78. 1887.

17. Weber M. *Economy and Society; an outline of interpretative sociology.* (Reprint). New York: Bedminister Press; 1968.

18. New South Wales. Votes and proceedings of the Legislative Council. Sydney: Government Printer; 1876.

19. Pyke-Lees W. *Centenary of the General Medical Council, 1858-1958.* London: General Medical Council; 1958.

20. Drucker S. The sickness of government. *The Public Interest.* 1969; 14:1-23.

21. Knight K. *The development of the public service in New South Wales from Responsible Government (1856) to the establishment of the Public Service Board.* [Doctoral]: University of Sydney; 1955.

22. Weber op cit.

23. New South Wales. Parliamentary debates 1:1 12/3/1880, pp1530-31.

24. Hilder E. *One hundred and twenty years of medical registration in New South Wales.* Sydney: New South Wales Medical Board; 1959.

25. New South Wales. Report of the Select Committee on the new constitution in New South Wales. . Sydney: Legislative Council; 1853. p. 119.

26. Parker RS. *The government of New South Wales.* St Lucia: University of Queensland Press; 1978.

27. Davis S. *The professsionalisation of medicine in N.S.W. 1870-1900* Ch.4 p.2. Sydney: University of New South Wales; 1983.

28. Lloyd. op cit.

CHAPTER 2 - *REFERENCES*

1. New South Wales. Parliamentary debates 1:1 12/3/1880, pp1530-31.
2. New South Wales. Parliamentary Debates 1:3:14/5/1880 p2327. 1880.
3. *Australasian Medical Gazette*. Quackery. 1873.
4. New South Wales. Parliamentary Debates, 1:3 14/5/1880 P2327 1880.
5. Pensabene T. *The rise of the medical practitioner in Victoria*. Canberra: Australian National University; 1980.
6. New South Wales. Parliamentary debates 5/8/1897. Sydney 1897 p. 2618.
7. New South Wales. Parliamentary debates 1897. p. 3658-60.
8. Lloyd P. *A social history of medicine; medical professionalisation in New South Wales, 1788-1950*. [Doctoral]. Sydney: University of New South Wales; 1993.
9. New South Wales. Parliamentary debates 21/3/1895. p. 4700-01.
10. Creed J. The Medical Practitioners' Bill. *The Australasian Medical Gazette*. 1900:113-4.
11. New South Wales Parliament. Select Committee inquiry. Sydney: NSW Government; 1887.
12. ibid p143.
13. *Australasian Medical Gazette*. Editorial. 1898.

CHAPTER 3 - *REFERENCES*

1. New South Wales. Journal of the Legislative Council 1856. p. 249-50.
2. Davis S. *The professionalisation of medicine in N.S.W. 1879-1900*. Sydney:[Masters] University of New South Wales; 1983.
3. New South Wales. Journal of the Legislative Council, 1887 (c) pp405-423. 1887.
4. Lloyd P. *A social history of medicine; medical professionalisation in*

New South Wales, 1788-1950. [Doctoral]. Sydney: University of New South Wales; 1993.

5. New South Wales. *Report of the Chief Medical Advisor to the Government.* Sydney: Government of New South Wales; 1897. p. 1061.

6. Willis E. (1991) *Medical dominance; the division of labour in Australian health care.* Sydney: Allen & Unwin.

7. New Zealand. Laws and Statutes. Wellington 1867. p. 407-14.

8. Fraenkel GW, (1994) *The Medical Board of South Australia 1884-94.* St Peters: Medical Board of South Australia.

9. Queensland. *Acts and statutes of Queensland.* 1911. pp. 2108-22.

10. Western Australia. *The Acts of the Parliament of Western Australia (1893) passed in the fifty-eighth year of the reign of her majesty queen Victoria during the first session f the second parliament of Western Australia.* Perth: Government Printer; 1894.

11. Starr M (1992). *The social transformation of American medicine* New York: Basic Books.

12. New South Wales. Parliamentary debates 6/7/1898 p.531.

13. New South Wales. Parliamentary Debates 1:105 18/9/1900 p2978.

14. Berlant J.(1975) *Profession and monopoly. A study of medicine in the United States and Great Britain.* Berkeley: University of California Press.

15. New South Wales. Parliamentary Debates 1:105 18/9/1900 p4524. 1900.

16. New South Wales. Parliamentary Debates Vol 106 1/11/1900, p4637. 1900.

17. Weekly Notes pp127-29, (1917).

CHAPTER 4 - *REFERENCES*

1. New South Wales. Report of the Director General of Public Health, New South Wales, for the year ended 31st December, 1913. Sydney, Government Printer, 1915.

2.   New South Wales. Report of the Director General of Public Health for 1938. Sydney: Government Printer; 1940 (b).

3.   Hilder E. (1959) *One hundred and twenty years of medical registration in New South Wales.* Sydney: New South Wales Medical Board.

4.   Haines G. (1997) *A history of the Pharmacy Board of New South Wales.* Sydney: The Pharmacy Board of New South Wales.

5.   New South Wales. The Statutes of New South Wales (of Practical Utility) Sydney: H.M. Cockshot, S.E. Lamb (eds); 1901.

6.   Anonymous. (1924) *History of the New South Wales Nurses' Registration Board.* Sydney: NSW Nurses' Registration Board;

7.   Optometry Board of New South Wales (1938). *The Optometry Board of New South Wales* pp643-53.

8.   New South Wales. Parliamentary debates 18/8/1963. p.4063.

9.   Parker RS. (1978) *The government of New South Wales.* St Lucia: University of Queensland Press.

10. Bagehot W. (1864) *The English constitution.* London: Collins.

11. Pensabene T. (1980) *The rise of the medical practitioner in Victoria.* Canberra: Australian National University. .

12. *Medical Journal of Australia.* Editorial. The NSW Medical Practitioners' Act. 1938.

13. New South Wales. Parliamentary debates 18/8/1938. p463.

14. New South Wales. (1998) *The New South Wales Parliamentary Record. From the first Council appointed August 11 1824 up to and including members elected to the 51st Parliament since the general election.* Sydney: Parliament of New South Wales.

15. New South Wales. Parliamentary debates 17/7/1938. pp407-15.

16. New South Wales. Parliamentary debates 30/11/1938. p3076.

CHAPTER 5 - *REFERENCES*

1.   Di Stefano V. (2006) *Holism and Complementary Medicine. Origins and principles.* Sydney: Allen & Unwin.

2. New South Wales. Parliamentary Debates 2:153 18/8/1938 pp1143-4.

3. Hunter T. Medical politics; decline in the hegemony of the Australian Medical Association. *Social Science and Medicine.* 1984; 18:973-80.

4. Lupton D. Doctors on the medical profession. *Sociology of Health and Illness.* 1997; 19:484-97.

5. Lloyd P. *A social history of medicine; medical professionalisation in New South Wales, 1788-1950.* [Doctoral]. Sydney: University of New South Wales; 1993.

6. McKay D. The Politics of Reaction, . In: Gardner H, editor. (1995) *The Politics of Health; the Australian Experience (2nd Ed).* Melbourne: Churchill Livingstone, pp344-70.

7. New South Wales. Parliamentary Debates, 3:45 27/3/1963 p3807

8. New South Wales. *Report of the Director General of Public Health for 1938.* Sydney: Government Printer; 1940 (b).

9. New South Wales. Board of Health. Minutes of proceedings 3 Jan 1897 - 11 April 1973.

10. Australian Medical Association Public Relations Committee. Report. 1962.

11. New South Wales. Parliamentary Debates 3:99 7/9/1972 p791.

12. Thomas David. Medical Autonomy and Peer Review in New South Wales [Doctoral]: University of Sydney; 2002.

13. Medical Registration Board of NSW. Annual Report. 1967. p4

14. Medical Registration Board NSW. Annual Report. 1972. p5.

15. Department of Health NSW. Role of the Complaints Unit. Complaints Unit Archives. File F/1; 1984.

16. Walton M. *Kept in the dark: Chelmsford, a case study of patients being denied information* [Masters]. Sydney: University of Sydney; 1990.

17. Illich I.(1976) *Medical nemesis: the expropriation of health:* London Calder & Boyars; 1

18. Taylor R. (1979) *Medicine out of control.* Melbourne: Sun Books.

19. Willis E. (1991) *Medical dominance; the division of labour in Australian health care.* Sydney, Allen & Unwin.

20. Le Fanu J. (1999) *The rise and fall of modern medicine.* London: Little Brown & Co.

21. Halpin D. (1974) Consumers Choice; 25 years of the Australian Consumers' Association. *Choice.*

22. Australian Consumers Association. Annual Report, 1980.

23. Bates, E. (1983) *Health systems and public scrutiny; Australia, Britain and the United States.* London: Croom Helm.

24. New South Wales. Parliamentary Debates, 3:78 12/3/1969, p4447

25. New South Wales Consumer Affairs Bureau. *Annual Report.* Sydney, 1972

26. New South Wales Consumer Affairs Bureau. *Annual Report.* Sydney 1980

27. Wilenski P.(1986) *Public Power and Public Administration.* Sydney: Hale & Ironmonger.

28. New South Wales. Parliamentary Debates 3:160 24/2/1981, p3975

29. New South Wales Law Reform Commission (1982). *Second report on the legal profession. Complaints, discipline and professional standards.* Sydney: The Commission.

30. Pirotta MV, Kotsirilos V, Farish S, Cohen, M. Complementary therapies: have they become accepted in general practice? *Medical Journal of Australia.* 2000; 172:February 2000.

31. Metherell M. Doctor seeks a better alternative. *The Australian.* 2010 May 29, 2010.

32. Baer H (2009). *Complementary medicine in Australia and New Zealand: its popularisation, legitimation and dilemmas.* Maleny, Verdant House.

33. Phelps K. AMA sees place for an alternative. *The Weekend Australian.* 2001.

34. Australian Medical Association. Complementary medicine.

Position Paper, 2002.

35. Australian Medical Association. Complementary medicine. Position Paper. 2012.

36. Spedding S. Regulation of conventional and complementary medicine - it is all in the evidence. *Medical Journal of Australia.* 2012; 196:682-3.

37. Dix A. Interview with author. 2008.

CHAPTER 6 - *REFERENCES*

1. Inglis B. (1964) *Fringe Medicine.* London: Faber and Faber; .

2. Alternative medicine. Merriam-Webster Dictionary, 2014.

3. Horin A. Alternative medicine. *National Times.* 1978:37-9.

4. Wardle J. Conference report: 10th international conference on herbal medicine. *Advances in Integrative Medicine.* 2017; 4:84-5.

5. Commonwealth of Australia (Webb Report). Report of the Committee of Inquiry into chiropractic, osteopathy, homeopathy and naturopathy. Canberra: AGPS; 1977. p. 143-61.

6. Baer H. The growing legitimation of complementary medicine in Australia; successes and dilemmas. *Australian Journal of Medical Herbalism.* 2008; 20:5-11.

7. Lloyd P, Lupton D, Wiesner D, Hasleton, S. Choosing alternative therapy; an exploratory study of sociodemographic characteristics and motivations of patients resident in Sydney. *Australian and New Zealand Journal of Public Health.* 17. June 1993, pp135-144.

8. Siapush M. Why do people favour alternative medicine? *Australian and New Zealand Journal of Public Health.* 1999; 23:266-71.

9. Rayner L, Easthope G. Postmodern consumption and alternative medications. *Journal of Sociology.* 2004; 37:157-76.

10. Boven R, Payne S, Sheehan M, Western J,. Current patients of alternative health care; a three-city study 1977.

11. Coulter I, Willis E. The rise and rise of complementary and

alternative medicine; a sociological perspective. *Medical Journal of Australia*. 2004; 189:587-9.

12. Wilkinson J, Simpson M. High use of complementary therapies in a New South Wales rural community. *Australian Journal of Rural Health*. 2001; 9:166-71.

13. Eastwood H. Why are Australian GPs using alternative medicine? Postmodernisation, consumerism and the shift towards holistic health. *Journal of Sociology*. 2000; 36:24.

14. Parker M. Two into one won't go; conceptual, clinical, ethical and legal impedimenta to the convergence of CAM and orthodox medicine. *Bioethical Inquiry*. 2007; 4:7 19.

15. Wiesner D. Alternative medicine. *Current Affairs Bulletin*. 1983; 60:4-17.

16. MacLennan, A. Taylor, A. Prevalence and cost of alternative medicine in Australia. *The Lancet*. 1996; 347:569-73.

17. MacLennan A. Perspectives on complementary and alternative medicines [Book Review]. *Cancer Forum*. 2012; 36:75.

18. Armstrong A, Thiebaut, Brown L. Australian adults use complementary and alternative medicine in the treatment of chronic illness: a national study. *Australian and New Zealand Journal of Public Health*. 2011; 35:384-90.

19. Reid R SA, Wardle J, Trubody A, Adams, A. Complementary medicine use by the Australian population; a critical mixed studies systematic review of utilisation, perceptions and factors associated with use. *BMC Alternative Medicine*. 2016; 16.

20. Von Conrady D, Bonney, A. Patterns of complementary and alternative medicine use and health literacy in general practice patients in urban and regional Australia. *Australian Family Physician*. 2017; 46:316-20.

21. Weir M, Wardle J, Marshall B, Archer E. Complementary and alternative medicine and consumer law. *Competition and Consumer Law Journal*. 2013; 21:85-110.

22. Advances in Integrative Medicine. Complementary and integrative medicine as a middle class medicine: busting the myth. *Advances in Integrative Medicine* 2017:1-2.

23. Willis E. Introduction: taking stock of medical dominance. *Health Sociology Review: the journal of the health section of the Australian Sociological Association.* 2006; 15:421-31.

24. Wardle J, Adams J, Magalhaes R, Sibbritt D. Distribution of complementary and alternative medicine (CAM) providers in rural New South Wales, Australia: a step towards explaining high CAM use in rural health? *Australian Journal of Rural Health.* 2011; 19:197-204.

25. Raszeja V, Jordens C, Kerridge I. Survey of practices and policies relating to the use of complementary and alternative medicines and therapies in New South Wales cancer services. *Internal Medicine Journal.* 2013; 43:84-8.

26. Qunlivan B. Feel better business. *Business Review Weekly* 6 April 2006.

27. Medical Journal of Australia. (W)holistic medicine. 1979; 2.

28. Lloyd P Lupton, D, Wiesner D, Hasleton S. Choosing alternative therapy; an exploratory study of sociodemographic characteristics and motives of of patients resident in Sydney. *Australian Journal of Public Health.* 1993; 17:133-44.

29. MacLennan A, D Taylor, A. Prevalence and cost of alternative medicine in Australia. *The Lancet.* 1996; 347:569-73.

30. Bensoussan A. Complementary medicine - where lies its appeal? *Medical Journal of Australia.* 1999; 170:247-8.

31. Spedding S. Regulation of conventional and complementary medicine - it is all in the evidence. *Medical Journal of Australia.* 2012; 196:682-3.

32. Wiesner D. (1983) *Professionalization under domination: the natural therapies in Australia.* Sydney: University of New South Wales [Doctoral];

33. Di Stefano V (2006). *Holism and Complementary Medicine. Origins and principles.* Sydney: Allen & Unwin.

34. Zaslawski C. Interview. with Author, 2017.

35. Zerbst V. Complementary medicine and academia. *Honi Soit.* August 29, 2016.

36. Harnett J. Evidence-based complementary medicines course begins in 2018. Sydney: University of Sydney Faculty of Pharmacy.; 2017.

CHAPTER 7 - *REFERENCES*

1. New South Wales. Parliamentary Debates 25/11/1971. 1971. p. 3336.

2. Willis E. Introduction: taking stock of medical dominance. *Health Sociology Review: the journal of the health section of the Australian Sociological Association.* 2006; 15:421-31.

3. Coburn D, Willis E. The medical profession. Knowledge, power, autonomy. In: Albrecht G, Fitzpatrick R, Scrimshaw S, editors. *Handbook of Social Studies in Health and Medicine.* London: Sage; 1998.

4. Devereaux E. History of chiropractic from a New South Wales perspective: a personal memoir. *ACO.* 1998; 7:68.

5. Baer H. *Complementary medicine in Australia and New Zealand. Its popularisation, legitimation and dilemmas* Maleny: Verdant 2009.

6. Commonwealth of Australia (Webb Report). Report of the Committee of Inquiry into chiropractic, osteopathy, homeopathy and naturopathy In: AGPS, editor. Canberra: AGPS; 1977. p. 143-61.

7. ibid p9.

8. Eastwood H. Why are Australian GPs using alternative medicine? Postmodernisation, consumerism and the shift towards holistic health. *Journal of Sociology.* 2000; 36:24.

9. Coulter I, Willis E. The rise and rise of complementary and alternative medicine; a sociological perspective. *Medical Journal of Australia.* 2004; 189:587-9.

10. Commonwealth of Australia. *Complememtary medicines in the Australian health system.* Report of the Parliamentary Secretary to the Minister for Health and Ageing Canberra: Department of Health and Ageing; 2003.

11. Commonwealth of Australia Complementary medicines in the Australian health system. Canberra: Expert committee on complementary medicines in the health system.; 2003. p. 147-8.

12. New South Wales. Regulation of complementary health practitioners. in Australia in:Complementary Therapies in Medicine. 10:1 March 2002.

13. Weir M. Regulation of complementary and alternative medicine practitioners: [Modalities of naturopathy, chiropractic, osteopathy, therapeutic massage therapy, traditional Chinese medicine (including Chinese herbal medicine and acupuncture), western herbal medicine, and homeopathy. Paper in: Regulating Health Practitioners. Freckelton, Ian (ed).]. *Law in Context.* 2006; 23:171-98.

14. Australian Government. Expert Committee on Complementary Medicines in the Health System, editor. Canberra: Department of Health Therapeutic Goods Administration; 2003.

15. ibid p143.

16. National Institute for Complementary Medicine. The National Institute of Complementary Medicine. In: NICM, editor. Sydney: Sydney; 2014.

17. NSW Ministry for Science and Medical Research. *Complementary medicine research:* a snapshot. Sydney 2005.

18. p143 *ibid.*

19. National Health and Medical Research Council. Complementary medicine gets a boost. Canberra: Australian government; 2008.

20. National Health and Medical Research Council. Major $640 million investment in Australia's world-leading medical research. Media Release December 2017. 2017.

21. National Press Club Speakers. Prof Warwick Anderson. *Australia's health - is research the best medicine?* April 15, 2015.

22. National Health and Medical Resource Council (2015) *Talking with your patients about complementary medicine – a resource for clinicians.* NHMRC Ref CAM001.

CHAPTER 8 - *REFERENCES*

1. Australian Health Ministers' Advisory Council. Options for regulation of unregistered health practitioners. 2013.

2. ibid.

3. Hewitt N. Interview with author. 1993.

4. New South Wales. Report of the Royal Commission into Deep Sleep Therapy. The Honourable Mr Acting Justice J.P. Slattery, Sydney: The Royal Commission.; 1990.

5. New South Wales Department for Health. Report of the Investigation Section of the Commonwealth Department of Health,. 1984. p. 6.

6. Complaints Unit. Annual report. 1985.

7. Complaints Unit. Annual Report. 1987.

8. Degeling, P Thomas D. Health policy. In: Laffin M PM, editor. *Reform and reversal. Lessons from the Coalition Government of New South Wales.* South Melbourne: Macmillan; 1995.

9. Jones A. *Sunday Telegraph.* 1993.

10. Selby H. Lawyers should support a public interest law centre. *Australian Law News.* 1992; 2.

11. Thomas D G. New South Wales: the Complaints Unit/Health Care Complaints Commission. In *Medicine called to account; health complaints mechanisms in Australisia.* Sydney: Graduate Management Programs, School of Public Health and Community Medicine, University of New South Wales; 2002. p. 15-30.

12. New South Wales Committee on the Health Care Complaints Commission. *Unregistered health practitioners. The adequacy and apropriateness of current mechanisms for resolving complaints.* Legislative Assembly of the Parliament of New South Wales; 1998.

13. Committee on the Health Care Complaints Commission Unregistered practitioners; the adequacy and appropriateness of current mechanisms for resolving complaints. Sydney: Legislative Assembly of NSW; 1998. p. 53.

14. New South Wales Committee on the Health Care Complaints Commission. History and Roles of the Committee on the Health Care Complaints Comiission 1994-2004. Sydney: Parliament of New South Wales; 2004. p. 9.

15. New South Wales Committee on the Health Care Complaints Commission. The Adequacy and Appropriateness of Current Mechanisms for Resolving Complaints. 1998.

16. Committee on the Health Care Complaints Commission. History and roles of the Committee on the Health Care Complaints Commission 1994-2004. 2004.

17. Committee on the Health Care Complaints Commission. Unregistered health practitioners. The adequacy and appropriateness of current mechanisms for resolving complaints. Sydney: Legislative Assembly of the Parliament of New South Wales; 1998.

18. Health Care Complaints Committee. Review of the 1998 report into 'Unregistered health practitioners; the adequacy and appropriateness of current mechanisms for resolving complaints'. Sydney 2006. p. 76.

19. Joint parliamentary committee inquiry into cosmetic service complaints. Submission by the Health Care Complaints Commission,. Sydney: Parliament of New South Wales; 2018. p. 3.

20. Wardle J. Holding unregistered health practitioners to account; an analysis of current regulatory and legislative approaches. *Journal of Law & Medicine.* 2014; 22:350-75.

21. Association ANT. https//:Australiannaturaltherapistsassociation.com.au.

22. Bye C. Lounge room drastic surgery. *Daily Telegraph.* 2018.

23. Bye C. It's time to knife cowboys. *Daily Telegraph.* 2018.

24. Health Care Complaints Commission of NSW. Statement of decision for Ian Pile. 2016.

25. Committee HCCC. Cosmetic health service complaints in New South Wales; submission by the Health Care Complaints Commission. Sydney: HCCC Parliamentary Committee; 2018.

26. Health Care Complaints Commission of NSW. Statement of

decision for Ms Pu Liu also known as Ms Mabel Liu. Sydney: Health Care Complaints Commission of NSW; 2016.

27. Joint Committee on the Health Care Complaints Commission. Cosmetic Health Service Complaints in New South Wales. In: Joint Committee on the Health Care Complaints Commission, editor. Sydney: The Committee; 2018. p. 128.

CHAPTER 9 - *REFERENCES*

1. Coulter I, Willis E. The rise and rise of complementary and alternative medicine, *Medical Journal of Australia* (180) 11, July 2004.

2. Shimadry B. New South Wales Department of Health. Letter to Dr D.G. Thomas, 2017.

3. https://www.skeptics.com.au/2017/11/19/2017-bent-spoon-to-nicm-skeptic-of-the-year-.

4. Harvey C. Don't duck the law by taking kids to quacks. *Sunday Telegraph*. 2016.

5. Vagg E. Leave facts out of the 'debate' about homeopathy. *The Conversation*. 2015.

6. Foley M. Leave facts out of 'debate' on homeopathy. *The Conversation*. 2015.

7. Musgrave I. So the NHMRC has found homeopathy doesn't work. Now how do we get the message across? *The Conversation*. 2015.

8. Freckleton I. Death by homeopathy; issues for civil, criminal and coronial law and for health service policy. *Journal of Law and Medicine*. 2012; 19:454-78.

9. Editorial. Is there a place for CAMS and traditional medicines in modern healthcare? *The Bitter Pill*. 2016.

10. Dana McCauley. Anger as uni cuts Chinese medicine degree. *Sydney Morning Herald*. 2019 25/07/2019.

11. Association Australian Homeopathic Association. https:www.yourhealthyourchoice.com.au. 2019.

12. Myers S, Xue C, Cohen M, Phelps K, Lewith, G. The legitimacy of academic complementary medicine. *Medical Journal of Australia.* 2012; 197:69-70.

13. Aubusson K. Homeopathic products stay on shelves. *Sydney Morning Herald.* 2018.

14. Australia Medical Board of Australia. Public consultation on clearer regulation of medical practitioners who provide complementary and unconventional medicine and emerging treatments. Melbourne: Medical Board of Australia; 2019.

15. McIntyre E Adams J, Foley H, Harnett J, Leach M, Reid R, Schloss J, Steel, A. Consultations with naturopaths and Western herbalists: prevalence of use and characteristics of users in Australia. *Journal of Alternative and Complementary Medicine.* 2019; 25:181-88.

16. Steel, A McIntyre E, Harnett J, Hope F, Adams J, Sibritt D, Wardle J, Frawley J. Complementary medicine use in the Australian population: Results of nationally representative cross-sectional servey. *Scientific Reports.* 2018; 8.

17. Cole-Adams K. Anaesthesia: the gift of oblivion. London: Text Publishing; 2017.

18. Carmody J. Some scientific reflections on possible mechanisms for general anaesthesia. https://wwwresearchgatenet/publication/243. 2018.

APPENDIX 1

AUSTRALIAN HEALTH PRACTITONERS' REGULATORY AGENCY (AHPRA) MEMBERSHIP

THE NATIONAL BOARDS

Aboriginal and Torres Strait Islander Health Practice Board of Australia*

Chinese Medicine Board of Australia

Chiropractic Board of Australia

Dental Board of Australia

Medical Board of Australia

Medical Radiation Practice Board of Australia

Nursing and Midwifery Board of Australia

Occupational Therapy Board of Australia

Optometry Board of Australia

Osteopathy Board of Australia

Para-medicine Board of Australia

Pharmacy Board of Australia

Physiotherapy Board of Australia

Podiatry Board of Australia

Psychology Board of Australia

*While Aboriginal and Torres Strait health practice is included in the 15 modalities listed above, that this is not based on Aboriginal and Torres Strait therapeutic practices but is focused on patient safety within the parameters of mainstream medicine and is seen to include elements of clinical and cultural safety as defined by Aboriginal and Torres Strait Islander peoples. (AHPRA communique, 9 November 2017)

APPENDIX 2

CODE OF CONDUCT FOR UNREGISTERED HEALTH PRACTITIONERS

Made under the Public Health Regulation 2012, Schedule 3 1

Definitions In this code of conduct: health practitioner and health service have the same meaning as in the Health Care Complaints Act 1993.

The Health Care Complaints Act 1993 defines those terms as follows: health practitioner means a natural person who provides a health service (whether or not the person is registered under the Health Practitioner Regulation National Law). Health service includes the following services, whether provided as public or private services: (a) medical, hospital, nursing and midwifery services, (b) dental services, (c) mental health services, (d) pharmaceutical services, (e) ambulance services, (f) community health services, (g) health education services, (h) welfare services necessary to implement any services referred to in paragraphs (a)–(g), (i) services provided in connection with Aboriginal and Torres Strait Islander health practices and medical radiation practices, (j) Chinese medicine, chiropractic, occupational therapy, optometry, osteopathy, physiotherapy, podiatry and psychology services, (j) optical dispensing, dietitian, massage therapy, naturopathy, acupuncture, speech therapy, audiology and audiometry services (k) services provided in other alternative health care fields, (l) forensic pathology services, (m) a service prescribed by the regulations as a health service for the purposes of the Health Care Complaints Act 1993. 2

Application of code of conduct This code of conduct applies to the provision of health services by: (a) health practitioners who are not subject to the scheme for registration under the Health Practitioner Regulation National Law (including de-registered health practitioners), and (b) health practitioners who are registered under the Health Practitioner Regulation National Law for the provision of health services and who provide health services that are unrelated to their registration. **Note.** Health practitioners may be subject to other requirements relating to the provision of health services to which this Code applies, including, for example, requirements imposed by Divisions 1 and 3 of Part 7 of the Act and by Part 4 of this Regulation.

Health practitioners to provide services in safe and ethical manner

1. A health practitioner must provide health services in a safe and ethical manner. (2) Without limiting subclause (1), health practitioners must comply with the following principles: (a) a health practitioner must maintain the necessary competence in his or her field of practice, (b) a health practitioner must not provide health care of a type that is outside his or her experience or training, (c) a health practitioner must not provide services that he or she is not qualified to provide, (d) a health practitioner must not use his or her possession of particular qualifications to mislead or deceive his or her clients as to his or her competence in his or her field of practice or ability to provide treatment, (e) a health practitioner must prescribe only treatments or appliances that serve the needs of the client, (f) a health practitioner must recognise the limitations of the treatment he or she can provide and refer clients to other competent health practitioners in appropriate circumstances, (g) a health practitioner must recommend to his or her clients that additional opinions and services be sought, where appropriate, (h) a health practitioner must assist his or her clients to find other appropriate health care professionals, if required and practicable, (i) a health practitioner must encourage his or her clients to inform their treating medical practitioner (if any) of the treatments they are receiving, (j) a health practitioner must have a sound understanding of any adverse interactions between the therapies and treatments he or she provides or prescribes and any other medications or treatments, whether prescribed or not, that the health practitioner is aware the client is taking or receiving, (k) a health practitioner must ensure that appropriate first aid is available to deal with any

misadventure during a client consultation, (1) a health practitioner must obtain appropriate emergency assistance (for example, from the Ambulance Service) in the event of any serious misadventure during a client consultation.

2. Health practitioners diagnosed with infectious medical condition A health practitioner who has been diagnosed with a medical condition that can be passed on to clients must ensure that he or she practises in a manner that does not put clients at risk. (2) Without limiting subclause (1), a health practitioner who has been diagnosed with a medical condition that can be passed on to clients should take and follow advice from an appropriate medical practitioner on the steps to be taken to modify his or her practice to avoid the possibility of transmitting that condition to clients.

Health practitioners not to make claims to cure certain serious illnesses

A health practitioner must not hold himself or herself out as qualified, able or willing to cure cancer or other terminal illnesses. A health practitioner may make a claim as to his or her ability or willingness to treat or alleviate the symptoms of those illnesses if that claim can be substantiated.

Health practitioners to adopt standard precautions for infection control

A health practitioner must adopt standard precautions for the control of infection in his or her practice. A health practitioner who carries out a skin penetration procedure must comply with the relevant provisions of this Regulation in relation to the carrying out of the procedure. *Note.* The Act defines skin penetration procedure as any procedure (whether medical or not) that involves skin penetration (such as acupuncture, tattooing, ear piercing or hair removal), and includes any procedure declared by the regulations to be a skin penetration procedure, but does not include: (a) any procedure carried out by a health practitioner registered under the Health Practitioner Regulation National Law, or by a person acting under the direction or supervision of a registered health practitioner, in the course of providing a health service, or (b) any procedure declared by the regulations not to be a skin penetration procedure.

Appropriate conduct in relation to treatment advice

A health practitioner must not attempt to dissuade clients from seeking or continuing with treatment by a registered medical practitioner. (2) A health practitioner must accept the right of his or her clients to make informed choices in relation to their health care. (3) A health practitioner should communicate and co-operate with colleagues and other health care practitioners and agencies in the best interests of their clients. (4) A health practitioner who has serious concerns about the treatment provided to any of his or her clients by another health practitioner must refer the matter to the Health Care Complaints Commission.

8. Health practitioners not to practise under influence or alcohol or drugs

A health practitioner must not practise under the influence of alcohol or unlawful drugs. (2) A health practitioner who is taking prescribed medication must obtain advice from the prescribing health practitioner on the impact of the medication on his or her ability to practice and must refrain from treating clients in circumstances where his or her ability is or may be impaired.

9. Health practitioners not to practice with certain physical or mental conditions

A health practitioner must not practise while suffering from a physical or mental impairment, disability, condition or disorder (including an addiction to alcohol or a drug, whether or not prescribed) that detrimentally affects, or is likely to detrimentally affect, his or her ability to practise or that places clients.

10. *Health practitioners not to financially exploit clients*

(1) A health practitioner must not accept financial inducements or gifts for referring clients to other health practitioners or to the suppliers of medications or therapeutic goods or devices. (2) A health practitioner must not offer financial inducements or gifts in return for client referrals from other health practitioners. (3) A health practitioner must not provide services and treatments to clients unless they are designed to maintain or improve the clients' health or wellbeing.

11. *Health practitioners required to have clinical basis for treatments*

A health practitioner must not diagnose or treat an illness or condition without an adequate clinical basis.

12. *Health practitioners not to misinform their clients*

(1) A health practitioner must not engage in any form of misinformation or misrepresentation in relation to the products or services he or she provides or as to his or her qualifications, training or professional affiliations. (2) a health practitioner must provide truthful information as to his or her qualifications, training or professional affiliations if asked for information about those matters by a client. (3) a health practitioner must not make claims, either directly or in advertising or promotional material, about the efficacy of treatment or services provided if those claims cannot be substantiated.

13. *Health practitioners not to engage in sexual or improper personal relationship with clients*

(1) a health practitioner must not engage in a sexual or other close personal relationship with a client. (2) before engaging in a sexual or other close personal relationship with a former client, a health practitioner must ensure that a suitable period of time has elapsed since the conclusion of their therapeutic relationship.

14. Health practitioners to comply with relevant privacy laws

A health practitioner must comply with the relevant legislation of the state or the commonwealth relating to his or her clients' health information, including the privacy act 1988 of the commonwealth and the health records and information privacy act 2002.

15. Health practitioners to keep appropriate records

A health practitioner must maintain accurate, legible and contemporaneous clinical records for each client consultation.

16. Health practitioners to keep appropriate insurance

A health practitioner should ensure that appropriate indemnity insurance arrangements are in place in relation to his or her practice.

17. Certain health practitioners to display code and other information

(1) A health practitioner must display a copy of each of the following documents at all premises where the health practitioner carries on his or her practice: (a) this code of conduct, (b) a document that gives information about the way in which clients may make a complaint to the health care complaints commission, being a document in a form approved by the secretary. (2) copies of those documents must be displayed in a position and manner that makes them easily visible to clients entering the relevant premises. (3) this clause does not apply to any of the following premises: (a) the premises of any body within the public health system (as defined in section 6 of the health services act 1997), (b) private health facilities (as defined in the private health facilities act 2007) (c) premises of the ambulance service of nsw (as defined in the health services act 1997), (d) premises of approved providers (within the meaning of the aged care act 1997 of the commonwealth).

18. Sale and supply of optical appliances

(1) A health practitioner must not sell or supply an optical appliance (other than cosmetic contact lenses) to a person unless he or she does so in accordance with a prescription from a person authorised to prescribe the optical appliance under section 122 of the health practitioner regulation national law. (2) a health practitioner must not sell or supply contact lenses to a person unless the health practitioner: (a) was licensed under the optical dispensers act 1963 immediately before its repeal, or (b) has a certificate iv in optical dispensing or an equivalent qualification. (3) a health practitioner who sells or supplies contact lenses to a person must provide the person with written information about the care, handling and wearing of contact lenses, including advice about possible adverse reactions to wearing contact lenses. (4) this clause does not apply to the sale or supply of the following: (a) hand-held magnifiers, (b) corrective lenses designed for use only in diving masks or swimming goggles, (c) ready made spectacles that: (i) are designed to alleviate the effects of presbyopia only, and (ii) comprise 2 lenses of equal power, being a power of plus one dioptre or more but not exceeding plus 3.5 dioptres. (5) in this clause: cosmetic contact lenses means contact lenses that are not designed to correct, remedy or relieve any refractive abnormality or defect of sight. optical appliance has the same meaning as it has in section 122 of the health practitioner regulation National Law.

CONCERNED ABOUT YOUR HEALTH CARE?

The Code of Conduct for unregistered health practitioners sets out what you can expect from your provider. If you are concerned about the health service that was provided to you or your next of kin, talk to the practitioner immediately. In most cases the health service provider will try to resolve them. If you are not satisfied with the provider's response, contact the Inquiry Service of the Health Care Complaints Commission on (02) 9219 7444 or toll free on 1800 043 159 for a confidential discussion. If your complaint is about sexual or physical assault or relates to the immediate health or safety of a person, you should contact the Commission immediately.

APPENDIX 3

EXAMPLES OF NEGATIVE REGULATION CASES INVESTIGATED BY THE HCCC

When cases are brought to the HCCC in terms of the Unregistered Practitioners Act, its investigations are as exhaustive and thorough as any conducted by the professional registration boards of the AHPRA. Two examples of such cases are cited by the HCCC to illustrate this point.

CASE 1

The first involved a herbalist who falsely claimed accreditation from a university and told a client with inoperable bowel and liver cancer that he could cure her within weeks. He was reluctant to tell her the ingredients of tablets he sold to her but which made her vomit, refused to give her a receipt for the payment he received and said it would be illegal to refund the $600 he had charged for two consultations when it became clear that his remedies were not working.

The patient died a year after first consulting the therapist, who was found by the HCCC investigation to have breached six of the clauses of the Code of Conduct. He was prohibited from further practice with any patient 'without the approval and oversight of the patient's general practitioner'. If the patient had no GP, the therapist was prohibited from 'prescribing or providing any herbal medicine to that client'.

CASE 2

Another complaint investigated by the HCCC was against one of the rapidly growing number of those whose 'business objective is primarily commercial and not curative or care orientated' might have seemed to be qualitatively different because it did not involve medications of any kind. However, it did involve medical issues, having been made by a complainant against a practitioner who in an advertisement had claimed to be a facial cosmetic surgeon able to perform a double eyelid-suturing procedure that would leave no bruising or scarring and have a 3-5 day recovery.

The investigators were told by the complainant that the procedure was carried out in a bedroom in the therapist's flat. The therapist demanded a payment of $1,500 before she commenced the procedure (although he later refunded this after the complainant expressed dissatisfaction with the outcome) which took close on seven hours to complete. The complainant asserted that her eyes had been seriously damaged by the procedure which had resulted in bruising, bleeding and scarring. The therapist had not worn surgical gloves while her two pet cats had wandered freely in an out of the room during the procedure.

After receiving a complaint, representatives of the HCCC, the Public Health Unit and the Pharmaceutical Regulatory Unit inspected Ms Liu's 'surgery'. They noted the absence of 'single use towels for drying hands, sterile gloves, appropriate sharps container, or appropriate surgical instrument sterilisation equipment.' At first the therapist claimed she had not performed cosmetic procedures on anyone but herself but later admitted that she had performed an eye-lid stitching procedure on one client.

The HCCC investigators found that she was not qualified or trained to perform even that procedure and that she had failed to exercise reasonable care and skill. As a result of these findings, the 'therapist' was banned by the HCCC from providing any cosmetic surgery or treatment for three years and permanently prohibited from providing treatments thereafter unless she could show that she had obtained qualifications to provide cosmetic surgery 'with reasonable care and skill'.

BIBLIOGRAPHY

ACADEMIC THESES

Davis S. *The professionalisation of medicine in N.S.W. 1870-1900* . (MA) University of New South Wales; 1983.

Knight K. *The development of the public service in New South Wales from Responsible Government (1856) to the establishment of the Public Service Board.* [PhD]: University of Sydney; 1955.

Lloyd P. *A social history of medicine; medical professionalisation in New South Wales, 1788-1950.* [PhD]. Sydney: University of New South Wales; 1993.

Thomas, D. *Medical Autonomy and Peer Review in New South Wales* (PhD) University of Sydney, 2002.

Walton, M. *Kept in the dark: Chelmsford: a case study of patients being denied information.* (MA) University of Sydney, 1990

Wiesner, D.M, *Professionalisation under Domination. The Natural Therapies in Australia.* As a research dissertation towards the degree of Doctor of Philosophy in the School of Sociology, University of New South Wales, Sydney, 1983.

BOOKS AND BOOK CHAPTERS

Baer, H. (2009) *Complementary Medicine in Australia and New Zealand. Its popularisation, legitimation and dilemmas.* Verdant House, Maleny, 2009

Bates, E. (1983) *Health systems and public scrutiny. Australia, Britain and the United States.* London, Croom Helm.

Bivins, R. (2012) *Alternative Medicine? A History.* Oxford, Oxford University Press

Bruck L. (1883) *The Australasian medical directory and hand-book* Sydney: Australian Medical Gazette.

Coburn D, Willis E (1998). The medical profession. Knowledge, power, autonomy. In Albrecht G, Scrimshaw S eds. *Handbook of Social Studies in Health and Medicine.* London, Sage.

Degeling P, Thomas D (1995). Health Policy, *in Reform and reversal. Lessons from the Coaltion Government of New South Wales.* Macmillan, South Melbourne.

Di Stefano, V. (2006) *Holism and Complementary Medicine. Origins and Principles.* Allen & Unwin, Sydney, 2006

Easthope, Gary. (2002) 'Alternative Medicine' *in* Germov, J. *Second opinion; an introduction to health sociology.* OUP, South Melbourne

Eastwood, H (2002) 'Globalisation. Complementary Medicine and Australian Health Policy: the Role of Consumerism' in *Health Policy in Australia* (2nd ed.) Gardner, H and Barraclough, S. eds. OUP, Oxford.

Gardner, H (ed) (1989) *The Politics of Health; the Australian experience.* Churchilll Livingstone, Melbourne.

Goldacre, B (2007) *Bad Science.* London, Fourth Estate

Halpin, D. (1974) *Consumers' choice. 25 years of the Australian Consumers' Association.* Choice, Sydney.

Hilder E. (1959) *One hundred and twenty years of medical registration in New South Wales.* Sydney: New South Wales Medical Board.

Johannessen, H, Lázár, I. (2006) *Multiple Medical Realities. Patients and Healers in Biomedical, Aternative and Traditional Medicine.* New York, Bergham Books.

Illich, I (1976) *Limits to medicine: medical nemesis; the expropriation of health.* London, Boyars.

Inglis, B. (1964) *Fringe Medicine.* London, Faber & Faber.

Le Fanu, J. (1999) *The rise and fall of modern medicine*. London, Abacus.

Macdonald, K. (1995) *The soociology of the professions*. London, Sage

McKay, D. (1995) The Politics of Reaction, *in* Gardner, H. *The politics of health: the Australian experience* (2nd ed) Melbourne, Churchill Livingstone.

Martyr, P. *Paradise of Quacks. An alterrnative history of medicine in Australia*. Macleay Press, Sydney, 2002

New South Wales. (1902) *The wealth and progress of New South Wales*. Sydney: W.A. Gulick Government Printer.

Parker, R.S. (1978) *The Government of New South Wales*. University of Queensland Press.

Porter R. (1989) *Health for sale; quackery in England, 1660-1850*. Manchester: Manchester University Press.

Taylor, R (1979) *Medicine out of control*. Sun Books, Melbourne

Thomas, D. (2002) (Ed) *Medicine called to account; health complaints mechanisms in Australasia*. Sydney, Graduate Management Programs, University of New South Wales.

Thomas, D (2002) Introductory overview *in Medicine called to account; health complaints mechanisms in Australia*. Sydney, Graduate Management Programs, University of New South Wales.

Wannan W. (1970)   *Folk medicine; a miscellany of old cures and remedies, superstitions, and old wives' tales having particular reference to Australia and the British Isles*. Melbourne: Hill of Content.

Weber M. (1968)   *Economy and Society; an outline of interpretative sociology*. (Reprint). New York: Bedminister Press.

Willis E. (1991) *Medical dominance; the division of labour in Australian health care*. Sydney: Allen & Unwin.

Willis, E. (1994) *Illness and social relations; issues in the sociology of health care.* Sydney, Allen & Unwin

Wootton, D (2006). *Bad Medicine. Doctors Doing Harm Since Hippocrates.* Oxford, OUP

JOURNAL ARTICLES

A

Advances in Integrative Medicine (2011). Complementary and integrative medicine as middle-class medicine: Busting the myth. *Advances in Integrative Medicine,*

Armstrong A, Thiébaut S, Brown L, Nepal B (2011). Australian adults use complementary and alternative medicine in the treatment of chronic illness: a national study. *Australian and New Zealand Journal of Public Health* 35:4 pp384-390

Australian Journal of Pharmacy [Editorial] (2014) The rise and rise of CAMS. 95:15/2/2014, pp44-6.

B

Baer, H. (2008). The growing legitimation of complementary medicine in Australia: successes and dilemmas. *Australian Journal of Medical Herbalism* 20(1) 2008 pp5-11.

Bensoussan, A (1999) Complementary medicine – where lies its appeal? Medical Journal of Australia: https://www.mja.co.au/journal 1999/170/6/complementary medicine.

Bonevski, B (2008) Complementary and alternative medicine in the news. *Issues,* 84 Sept 2008 pp 17-19

Bonevski B, Wilson A, Henry D (2008). An analysis of news media covererage of complementary and alternative medicine. http://journals.plos.org/plosone/article?id=10.1371/journal.pone.0002406

Bowditch, P. (2004) Quackery down under. Text of a presentation given by Peter Bowditch on January 16, 2004, to the Amazing Meeting 2 in Las Vegas http://ratings.com/soles/comment/tam2.htm

Boyce, R. (2006). Emerging from the shadow of medicine; allied health as a 'profession community' subculture. *Health Sociology Review. The Journal of the Australian Sociological Association.* 15:5 pp 520-534

Boven R, Payne S, Sheehan M, Western J (1977). Current patients of alternative health care: a three-city study. *The Australian Journal of Pharmacy:* 93:66-8.

Braun, L. (2014). The evidence is food for thought. *The Australian Journal of Pharmacy* Vol 95, 2014 pp22-4.

C

Chan J, Chan J (2000). Medicine for the millenium; the challenge of postmodernism. *Medical Journal of Australia* 172:7 332-334.

Chiropractic Journal of Australia (2012) Commentary: Quo Vadis? 42:2 pp72-3.

Complementary Medicines Australia (2014) *Complementary Healthcare Council of Australia. 2014 Federal pre-budget submission.* www.chc.org.au

Coulter I, Willis E (2004).. The rise and rise of complementary and alternative medicine; a sociological perspective. *Medical Journal of Australia.* 189:587-9.

D

Del Mar C. (2002) From quackery to evidence-based medicine. *Complementary Medicine.* July/August 2002.

Devereaux E. (1998), A history of chiropractic from a New South Wales Perspective (1969-1982). "A personal memoir". *ACO* 7:2, pp 68-79.

Devereaux E. (2012) Current chiropractic status in Australia: manpower and research needs. Commentary. *Chiropractic Journal of Australia*. 42:2 June 2012: 68-71

Drucker S.(1969). The sickness of government. *The Public Interest*. 1969; 14:1-23.

Dunne A, Phillips C. (2010) Complementary and alternative medicine. Representation in popular magazines. *Australian Physician* 31/9 pp671-3

Dwyer, J: Welcome from the President of Friends of Science in Medicine. http://www.scienceinmedicine.org.au 24/06/2015

E

Eastwood, H (2000) Why are Australian GPs using alternative medicine? Postmodernism, consumerism and the shift towards holistic health. *Journal of Sociology*, 26:2, pp133-156.

Ernst, Edzard (2015). Open letter to Prof Bruce Robinson from Prof Edzard Ernst. http://www.scienceinmedicine.org.au 24/06/2015

Ernst, Edzard. (2016). Integrative medicine; more than the promotion of unproven treatments? *Medical Journal of Australia*.204 (5):174.

F

Farley, L. (2014). The rise and rise of CAMS. *The Australian Journal of Pharmacy*. Vol 95 pp44-46.

Foley, M. 'Holistic' dentistry: more poppycock than panacea? *The Conversation*. http://theconversation.com/holistic-dentisry-more-poppycock-than-panacea-41177?

Fontanarosa, P (2001). Publication of complementary and alternative medicine research in mainstream biomedical journals. *Journal of Alternative and Complementary Medicine*. Vol 7, Supplement 1, 2001, pp s139-S143

Freckleton, I (2012). Death by homeopathy; issues for civil, criminal and coronial law for health service policy. *Journal of Law and Medicine*, 19:454-78

Freckleton, I. (2013) The emergence and evolution of health law *Law in Context*, 29:2, pp74-78

Freckleton, I. (2013) Legal implications for complementary medicine practitioners of the New South Wales Practitioner Code of Conduct. *Journal of Law and Medicine*. 734:20 pp1-11

Freckleton I. (2008) Regulating the unregistered. *Journal of Law and Medicine*, 16:413-8

Friends of Science in Medicine *The Bitter Pill*

What is 'good science' in medicine? 8/03/2016

How do CAM practitioners plan to expand their influence in healthcare?

Is there a place for CAMS and traditional medicines in modern healthcare?

"Alternative" health courses in Australian Universities

G

Georgetown Law Library. Complementary and alternative medicine research guide: http://www.law.georgetown.edu/library/research/guides/camedicinee.cfm.

Godfrey K, (2005) New GP network will integrate conventional and complementary medicine. *British MedicaL Journal*. 331, 22/10/2005 p924

H

Harvey, K. (2008) Australian complementary medicine regulation; time for reform! *Health Issues*, Issue 95, Winter 2008 pp18-22

Harvey K (2009) A review of proposals to reform the regulation of complementary medicines. *Australian Health Review*, 33:2, 279-287

Harvey, K. (2014) Don't believe the hype – your complementary medicines are unlikely to deliver. 14/12/2014,

Harvey, K. (2015) Kids smart dumb ads: consumers complain of misleading claims. 27/5/2015

Harvey K, Korczrak V, Marron L, Newgreen D. (2008). Commercialism, choice and consumer protection: regulation of complementary medicines in Australia. *Medical Journal of Australia* 188 (1) 21-5.

Holden, S. (2015) Oh, the uncertainty, how do we cope? *The Conversation*. September 10, 2015.

Hollenberg D, Muzzin L (2010). Epistemological challenges to integrative medicine: an anti-colonial perspective on the combination of complementary/alternative medicine with biomedicine. *Health Sociology Review* 19:1 pp34-56.

House, W. (2015) Holistic healthcare today. http//www.bhma.org/pages/aboutholistic-healthcare.php

Hilbers J, Lewis C (2013). Complementary health therapies; moving towards and integrated health model. *Collegian* 20:51-60

Hunter, J, Corcoran K, Phelps K, Leeder S (2012) The challenges of establishing an integrative medicine primary care clinic in Sydney, Australia. *The Journal of Alternative and Complementary Medicine* 18:11 pp1008-1013.

Hunter, T. (1980) Pressure groups and the Australian political process: the case of the Australian Medical Association. *Journal of Commonwealth and Comparative Politics*, pp191-206.

Hunter, T. (1984) Medical politics: decline in the hegemony of the Australian Medical Association, 18:11 *Medical Politics* pp 973-980

I

Ieraci, S. The burden of scientific proof. http://www.mja.com.au/insight/2013/21sue-ieraci-burden-scientific-proof.

Ieraci, S. "Alternative" is not a compliment. There is no such thing as "CAM", only medicine, complementary therapy and scam. *Australian Science,* June 2015

K

Kam, K. (2012) What is integrative medicine? Experts explore new ways to treat the mind, body, and spirit – all at the same time. http://www.webmd.com/a-to-z ideas/features/alternative-medicine-integrative-medicine.

Kune R, Kune G (2007), Mainstream medicine versus complementary and alternative medicine in the witness box: resolving the clash of ideologies. *Journal of Law and Medicine.* 14. Pp 425-432

L

Larsen, H (2002). Complementary medicine: why so popular? File:///A1/hyperlinks/Alterntive Medicine Why so popular.htm

Leach MJ, McIntyre E, Frawley. (2014) Characteristics of the Australian complementary and alternative medicine (CAM) workforce. *Australian Journal of Herbal Medicine,* 26(2) pp 58-65

Levy D, Gadd B. (2012). Epistemology and the ethics of homeopathy: a response to Freckleton. *Journal of Law and Medicine* 19:699.

Litscher G. (2014) No, there Is no conclusive scientific evidence for visualisation of meridians at the moment. *Journal of Alternative and Complementary Medicine* 20:3 pp215-216.

Lloyd, P, Lupton, D, Wiesner, D, Hasleton, S. (1993) Choosing alternative therapy: an exploratory stury of sociodemographic characteristics and motives of patients resident in Sydney. *Australian Journal of Public Health* 17:2.

Locke, S. How to debunk false beliefs without having it backfire. http://www.vox.com/2014/12/22/7433899/debunk-how-to

Lupton, D (1997). Doctors on the medical profession. *Sociology of Health and Illness,* 19:4 pp480-497.

M

Marron, L. "Integrative medicine" has no place in universities. *Australian Science,* July / August 2015

MacLennan, A, Morrison, R. (2012) Tertiary institutions should not offer pseudoscientific medical courses. *Medical Journal of Australia.* 198 (4) 225-226.

MacLennan A, Taylor A, Wilson, D (1996), Prevalence and cost of alternative medicine in Australia. *The Lancet,* 347, pp 569-573.

MacLennan A, Wilson D, Taylor, A. (2002) The escalating cost and prevalence of alternative medicine. *Preventative Medicine,* 35, 166-173.

McCabe, P (2005). Complementary and alternative medicine in Australia: a contemporary overview. *Complementary Therapies in Clinical Practice,* 11, 25-31.

McIntyre E, Adams , Foley H, Harnett J, Leach M, Reid R, Schloss, J, Steel A (2019) Consultations with Naturopaths and Western Herbalists; Prevalence and Characteristics of Users in Australia. *The Journal of Alternative and Complementary Medicine,* Vol 25:2, 20/2/2019

Medical Journal of Australia. The NSW Medical Practitioners' Act. [Editorial] *Medical Journal of Australia.* 1938.

Medew J. Alternative medicine crackdown. http://www.smh.com.au / federal- / political-news / alternative-medicine-crackdown-20120313-1 / uyw.htm

Medew, J. Push to rid universities of alternative medicine. http:// www.theage.com.au / national / health / push-to-rid-universities-of-alternative- medicine. 11 / 12 / 2012

Medical Journal of Australia. (Editorial) (W)holistic medicine, 1979: 2:467

Medical Journal of Australia. The NSW Medical Practitioners' Act. (Editorial) .

Micozzi, M. (1995). Alternative and complementary medicine; part of human heritage. (1995) *The Journal of Alternative and Complementary Medicine*, 1/1/1995. pp1-3.

Mitchell, D. (2008) The broad church of medical acupuncture. *Complementary Medicine*. Jan/Feb 2008 p20.

Musgrave, I. (2015) So, the NHMRC has found homeopathy doesn't work. Now how do we get this message across? *The Conversation*, 13/3/2015

Myers S, Xue, C, Cohen M, Phelps, K, Lewith G.(2012) The legitimacy of academic complementary medicine. *Medical Journal of Australia*,   197 (2) 69-70.

N

Niemetzow, R. (2013) Basic science: mysteries and mechanisms of acupuncture. *Medical Acupuncture* 25:2.

O

O'Brien, K. (2002) Commentary on C Zaslawski and S Davis, 'The ethics of complementary and alternative medicine research'. *Monash Bioethics Review*, 24:3 pp 62-66.

Olver, I (2011) Overview of complementary and alternative medicine. *Cancer Forum*. 35 (1) 2011 pp3-5.

O'Neill A, Willis E. (1994) Chiropractic and the politics of health care. *Australian Journal of Public Health*, 18:3, pp 325-331

P

Palmer, D. (2014) Explainer: what is postmodernism? *The Conversation*, 3/1/2014

Parker, M. (2007) Two into one won't go: conceptual, clinical, ethical and legal impediments to the convergence of CAM and orthodox medicine. *Bioethical Inquiry* 4:7-19

Pirri C (2011) Integrating complementary and conventional medicine *Cancer Forum* 36:1 pp31-9

Pirotta M, Cohen M, Kotsirilos V, Farish S (2000). Complementary therapies: have they become accepted in general practice? *Medical Journal of Australia*, 3:172, 7/2 2000, pp105-109

Q

Quinlivan, D. (2006) Feel better business. *Business Review Weekly*, April, 2006, p6

R

Raszeja, V.M., Jordens C, Kerridge I. (2013). Survey of practices and policies relating to the use of complementary and alternative medicines and therapies in New South Wales cancer services. *Internal Medicine Journal* 43, pp 84-89.

Rayner L, Easthope G. (2004) Postmodern consumption and alternative medications. *Journal of Sociology*, 37:2, pp157-176.

Reid R, Steel A, Wardle J, Trubody A, Adams J. (2016). Complementary medicine use by the Australian population: a critical mixed studies systematic review of utilisation, perceptions and factors associated with use. *Biomed Central. Complementary and Alternative Medicine Series – open, inclusive and trusted.* 2016 16:176

Robotin M, Penman A. (2006) Viewpoint: integrating complementary therapies into mainstream cancer care: which way forward? *Medical Journal of Australia* 185:7 pp 377-379.

S

Sarris, Jerome. (2012) Current challenges in appraising complementary medicine evidence. *Medical Journal of Australia* 196 (5) 310-311

Scholefield, A. (2017) Alternative medicine gets bent spoon award. https://www.medicalobserver.com.au

Schulz, E.N. Pseudoscience and conspiracy theory are not victimless crimes against science. 4/6/2015

Siapush, M. (1999) Why do people favour alternative medicine?

Australian and New Zealand Journal of Public Health. 23:266-71

Spedding, S (2012) Regulation of conventional and complementary medicine – it is all in the evidence. *Medical Journal of Australia* 196 (11) pp683-3

T

Tran, A. (2006). The regulation of traditional Chinese medicine practitioners in Australia. *The Journal of Law and Medicine.* 13:352

V

Vagg, Michael. Leave 'facts' out of the debate about homeopathy. *The Conversation,* 23/6/2015

Van Velden, D. The bio-, psycho-, social approach to health and disease. http//wwww.sun.as.za/stellmesd/docs/0108.doc

Voyce, M. (1994). Regulating alternative health. *Alternative Law Journal* 19:3, pp 132-138

W

Wardle, J. (2016) Defining deviation: the peer professional opinion defence and its relationship to scope expansion and emerging non-medical health professions. *Journal of Law and Medicine* 23 662-667.

Wardle J (2014) Holding unregistered health practitioners to account: an analysis of current regulatory and legislative approaches. *Journal of Law and Medicine* 22:350 pp 350-375.

Wardle J, Adams J, Margalhäes R, Sibbritt D. (2011) Distribution of complementary and alternative medicine (CAM) providers in New South Wales, Australia. A step towards explaining high CAM use in rural health? *Australian Journal of Rural Health* 19:4, pp197-204.

Wardle J, Sibritt D, Adams J. The interface with naturopathy in rural primary health care; a survey or referral practices of general practitioners in rural and regional New South Wales (2014) *BMC Alternative Medicine.* 14:238.

Wardle J, Sibbritt, Broom A, Steel, Adams J. (2016). Is health practitioner regulation keeping pace with the changing practitioner and health-care landscape.? An Australian perspective. *Frontiers in Public Health,* Vol 4, Article 91. Pp1-5.

Weir, M (2013). Legal implications for complementary medicine practitioners of the New South Wales Practitioner Code of Conduct. *Journal of Law and Medicine.* 22: 350-75.

Weir, M (2005) Regulation of complementary and alternative medicine practitioners. Paper in *Regulating Health Practitioners.* Freckleton, I (ed) *Law in Context,* 23:2 pp171-199.

Weir M, Wardle J, Marshall B, Archer E (2013) Complementary and alternative medicine and consumer law. *Competition and Consumer Law Journal* 2013:21:85-110 .

Wiesner, D. Alternative medicine.(1983) *Current Affairs Bulletin.* 60:4-17

Willis, E. (2006) Introduction: taking stock of medical dominance. *Health Sociology Review,* 15, Issue 5 pp 421-431.

Wilkinson J, Simpson M. (2001) High use of complementary therapies in a New South Wales rural community. *Australian Journal of Rural Health,* 9: pp166-171

Wolpe P (1985). The maintenance of professional authority: acupuncture and the American physician. *Social Problems,* 32:5, pp409-422

Woodhead, M. (2015) Fines will not stop quacks, say homeopathy critics. *Australian Doctor.* 14/10/2015.

Wooton, J, (1997) Directory of databases for research into alternative and complementary medicine. *The Journal of Alternative and Complementary Medicine.* Vo; 3:2, pp179-190

X

Xue C, Zhang L, Lin V, Story D. (2006) The use of complementary and alternative medicine in Australia. *Health Issues* No 88, pp 12-16

Xue C, Zhang A, Greenwood K, Lin V, Story, D. (2010) *The Journal of Alternative and Complementary Medicine.* 16:3 pp301-312

Y

Young, J.H, (1998) The development of the Office of Alternative Medicine in the National Institutes of Health, 1991-96. *Bulletin of the History of Medicine* 72:2 279-298

Z

Zhang T, M ay B, Yang A, Xue C. Zhang Z. (1995) Integrating acupuncture with the Australian health care system. *Issues (South Melbourne,* 84, pp38-42

Zaslawski C. Davis S. (2002) The ethics of complementary and alternative medicine research: a case study of Traditional Chinese Medicine at the University of Technology, Sydney. *Monash Bioethics Review,* 24:3 52-61

Zhu X, Carlton A, Bensoussan A (2009) Development in and challenge for traditional Chinese medicine in Australia.*The Journal of Alternative and Complementary Medicine.* 15:6 pp685-688

GOVERNMENT DOCUMENTS/PUBLICATIONS

Commonwealth of Australia. (1977) (Webb Report) Report of the Committee of Inquiry into chiropractic, osteopathy, homeopathy and naturopathy. Canberra, AGPS.

Commonwealth of Australia. (2003) Expert Committee on complementary medicines in the Australian health system. Canberra, Department of Health and Ageing. Therapeutic Goods Administration.

Commonwealth of Australia. (2013) Health Ministers' Advisory Council. Options for regulation of unregistered health practitioners.

National Institute for Complementary Medicine.(2014) The National Institute for Complementary Medicine, Sydney

National Health and Medical Research Council (2008). Complementary medicine gets a boost. Canberra, AGPS

National Health and Medical Research Council (March 2015) NHMRC statement on homeopathy. Canberra, AGPS

New South Wales. Board of Health. Minutes of proceedings 3/1/1897-11/4/1973

New South Wales. Board of Health. Minutes of proceedings 1973.

New South Wales. Department of Health. Complaints Unit. Annual Report, 1985

New South Wales. Department of Health. Complaints Unit. Annual Report, 1987

New South Wales Committee on the Health Care Complaints Commission. *Unregistered health practitioners. The adequacy and appropriateness of current mechanisms for resolving complaints.* Legislative Assembly of the Parliament of New South Wales, 1998.

New South Wales Committee on the Health Care Complaints Commission. *History and Roles of the Committee on the Health Care Complaints commission* 1994-2004.

New South Wales Committee on the Health Care Complaints Commission. *Review of the 1998 report into 'Unregistered health practitioners; the adequqcy and apropriateneess of current mechanisms for resolving complaints.* Sydney, 2006.

New South Wales Consumer Affairs Bureau. Annual Report, 1972

New South Wales Department of Health. Role of the Complaints Unit. Complaints Unit archives. File F/1:1984

New South Wales Department of Health. (2002) Regulation of complementary health practitioners. Sydney.

New South Wales Health Care Complaints Commission. Statement of decision for Mr Ian Pile, 2016.

New South Wales Health Care Complaints Commission. Statement of decision for Ms Pu Lie also known as Ms Mabel Liu, 2016

New South Wales. (2018) *Joint Committee inquiry into cosmetic health service complaints.* Submission by the Health Care Complaints Commission. Sydney, Parliament of New South Wales

New South Wales Health Care Complaints Commission. Annual Report, 2009

New South Wales Law Reform Commission. *Second report on the legal profession. Complaints, discipline and professional standards.* Sydney. The Commission, 1982.

New South Wales Medical Registration Board. Annual Report. 1967.

New South Wales Medical Registration Board. Annual Report. 1972.

New South Wales Ministry for Science and Medical Research. Complementary medicine research; a snapshot. 2005

New South Wales. Report from the Committee on the Medical Practice Bill with the minutes of evidence. Sydney: The Legislative Council; 1838.

New South Wales. Report of the Royal Commission into Deep Sleep Therapy. The Honourable Mr Justice J.P. Slattery. Sydney, the Royal Commission. 1990

New South Wales. Report of the Director-General of Public Health for 1938. (1940b)

New South Wales Report of the Select Committee on the new constitution in New South Wales. . Sydney: Legislative Council; 1853. p119.

New South Wales. Votes and proceedings of the Legislative Council. Sydney: Government Printer; 1876.

New South Wales. Parliamentary debates 1:1 12/3/1880, pp1530-31.

New South Wales. Parliamentary Debates 1:3:14/5/1880 p2327.

New South Wales. Parliamentary Debates 1887(a), p78. 1887

New South Wales. Parliamentary debates 21/3/1895. 1895. p. 4700-01.

New South Wales. Parliamentary debates 5/8/1897 p.2618.

New South Wales. Parliamentary debates 22/10/1897 p.3658-60.

New South Wales. Parliamentary debates 18/8/1938. 1938. p. 463.

New South Wales. Parliamentary debates 17/7/1938. 1938. p. 407-15; p. 643-53.

New South Wales. Parliamentary debates 18/8/1938. 1938. p. 463.

New South Wales. Parliamentary Debates 2:153 18/8/1938 pp1143-4. 1938.

New South Wales Parliamentary debates 30/11/1938. Sydney: New South Wales; 1938. p. 3076.

New South Wales. Parliamentary Debates 3:99 7/9/1972, p791

New South Wales. Parliamentary Debates 3:160 24/2/1981 p3975

New South Wales. The Statutes of New South Wales (of Practical Utility) Sydney: H.M. Cockshot, S.E. Lamb (eds); 1901.

New South Wales. *The wealth and progress of New South Wales.* Sydney: W.A. Gulick Government Printer; 1902.

New South Wales. Report of the Director General of Public Health, New South Wales, for the year ended 31st December, 1913. 1915.

New South Wales. Report of the Director General of Public Health for 1938. Sydney: Government Printer; 1940 (b).

New South Wales Report of the Select Committee on the new

constitution in New South Wales. Sydney: Legislative Council; 1853. p. 119.

New South Wales. Votes and proceedings of the Legislative Council. Sydney: Government Printer; 1876.

New South Wales. (1990). *Report of the Royal Commission into Deep Sleep Therapy/The Honourable Mr Acting Justice J.P. Slattery, Royal Commission.* Sydney: The Royal Commission.

New South Wales Parliament. Select Committee inquiry. Sydney: NSW Government; 1887.

National Health and Medical Research Council. Talking with your patients about Complementary Medicine. (2014) A resource for clinicians. NHMRC Ref CAM 001

LEGAL CASES CITED

Allinson v. General Council of Medical Registration and Education [1894] 1 QB

Clune vs Medical Board [1917] 314. *Weekly Notes* (NSW) 127

NEWSPAPER ARTICLES/MEDIA RELEASES

Alexander, H. (2017) Vitamin mogul donates $10m to university. *Sydney Morning Herald,* 12/4/2017

Alexander H, Phillips N. Alternative medicine or false hope? *The Sun Herald,* 31/5/2015, p15

Buchanan, M 29/08/2001. A natural high. *Sydney Morning Herald, My career supplement* 29/08/2001, p4.

Bye, C. Lounge room drastic surgery, *Daily Telegraph*2018

Bye, C. It's time to knife cowboys. *Daily Telegraph, 2018*

Commonwealth of Australia. Australian Bureau of Statistics (2008) Broadband, complementary health therapies and mortgages all on the up. 4102.0 Australian Social Trends, 2008. Media release.

Australian Bureau of Statistics (2008) Complementary therapies. Australian Social Trends 2008 4102.0. Media release

Harvey, Claire. 12/7/2015 Don't duck the law by taking kids to quacks. *Sunday Telegraph. p33*

Complementary Medicines Australia (2014) The five fundamental flaws of the NHMRC homeopathy review. 15/12/2014

Harnett, J (2017). Evidence-based complementary medicine course begins in 2018. University of Sydney Faculty of Pharmacy, 2017

Horin, A. (1978) Alternative medicine. *National Times*

Leser, D (2016) The medicine man. Dec 20, 2014 *Sydney Morning Herald Good Weekend* pp13-15

Macgregor, J. (2002)Holistic asks mainstream to take a complement. (2002) *Sydney Morning Herald,* 2/5/2002

Macken, Julie. A healthy alternative. 2/3/1999

Metherell, M.(2010) Doctor seeks a better alternative. Serious illness makes Kerryn Phelps rethink her approach. *The Australian,* May 2010

National Health and Medical Research Council (2017). Major $640 million investment in Australia's world leading medical research. Media Release, December 2017.

Parnell, Sean. (2015) Natural therapy cover risk to private health rebate. *The Australian 3/1/2015*

Quinlivan, B. ((2006) Profile Marcus Blackmore, Executive Chairman, Blackmores. The doyen of complementary health care believes that people should take more. *Business Review Weekly* 8/4/2008, P32

Ragg, M. Good medicine. *The Australian*, 11/11/1999, p13

Shoebridge, Neil. (1993) Health becomes a holistic market. *Business Review weekly*, 10/12/1993, p77

Singh, L. Feb 6-7, 2016. High wire support. *Sydney Morning Herald News Review.* p7

Urban E. (2015) China trade deal just the tnoic for vitamin maker Blackmores. *The Australian Financial Review* 22/11/2015, p14

University of Sydney (2017) Evidence-based complementary medicines course begin in 2018. Media Release.

Zerbst, V (2016) Complementary medicine and academia. *Honi Soit,* 29/9/2016 pp 1-2

ORGANISATIONS

New South Wales Consumer Affairs Bureau. *Annual Report.* Sydney1972.

Australian Consumers' Association. (1980) Annual Report incorporating ACA newsletter for ordinary members

Australian Medical Association. Public Relations Committee Report, 1962

POSITION PAPERS

Australian Medical Association. Position Paper: Complementary medicine. 2002.

Australian Medical Association. Position Paper. Complementary medicine. Position Paper. 2012.

National Health and Medical Research Council. (2014) Talking with our patients about complementary medicine - a resource of clinicians. NHMRCRef CAM001. 2004.

RACGP/AIMA (2004) Complementary medicine. Joint position statement of the RACGP and AIMA

Author bio

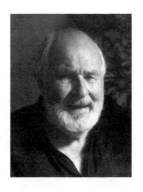 Dr David Thomas has never seen himself as anything but an 'opportunistic author' who launches into new literary projects only when he comes across subjects and issues which demand to be written up in book form. Such was the case when researching for his doctorate in the University of Sydney, he was surprised to discover the ferocity of the clash between supporters of orthodox medical practice and those who subscribed to complementary/alternative medicine in the State of New South Wales. The story of that clash, evident in the earliest records of medical practice in the State right up to the present, he saw as something worth adding to its historical tapestry. His early career in journalism in his native South Africa as well as in Australia, and also his teaching experience in the fields of politics, sociology and various health fields in several Australian universities, most particularly in the School of Public Health and Community Medicine (now in the process of being renamed Population Health) in the Medical Faculty of the University of New South Wales, equipped him well to undertake this current venture. He has been retired for a number of years but still holds the status of Honorary Senior Lecturer in the School of Population Health in the Medical Faculty.